"As a manager, there is nothing more frustrating than having a player out due to injury. I feel privileged to have Dr. Ahmad and his talented group of medical professionals taking care of our athletes each and every day. *Play Ball* does an exceptional job of providing the knowledge of our nation's top sports medicine specialists and delivering it in a way that makes it easy to follow, understand, and absorb. This book serves as a go-to guide, ensuring that athletes at all levels and abilities receive the same access to medical advice as our professionals."—*Joe Girardi, former manager of the NY Yankees*

"Whether you're working with youngster ball players or Cy Young Award Winners, the only way to mitigate the risk of injury is to truly understand the unique demands a sport puts on an athlete's body. In *Play Ball*, Ahmad and Gallucci present a thorough and easy-to-follow blueprint for keeping players healthy over the course of the season and performing at their peak. It's a must-read for personal trainers and coaches alike."—*Mickey Brueckner NASM-CPT, CSCS, FMS, founder and CEO, ANNEX Sports Performance Center*

"We now live in an era in amateur sports where early specialization and professional training have become the norm. Constant repetition, high intensity training, and overemphasized competition have led to an overwhelming number of overuse injuries, especially in the game of baseball. *Play Ball* sheds light on the prevention, occurrence, proper treatment, and rehabilitation of injuries associated with playing baseball."—*Mike Sheppard Jr., Head Baseball Coach, Seton Hall Prep*

"The Yogi Berra Museum & Learning Center is committed to sustaining Yogi's vision of youth sports as a unique vehicle for some of life's most important lessons, such as the value of perseverance, teamwork, and respect for others. What's clear is that young people won't benefit from sports if they are too injured to play. *Play Ball* provides a comprehensive and accessible guide to keeping a new generation of athletes in top form, no matter their skill level, so that our kids can experience the full range of positive values sports experiences can instill, both on the field and off."—*Eve Schaenen, Executive Director, Yogi Berra Museum & Learning Center*

"Throughout my tenure as a professional baseball player, I have seen my fair share of injuries, many of which could have been prevented. *Play Ball* does an exceptional job of giving a true understanding of sports medicine knowledge, written and executed in a way that makes it easy to follow, understand, and implement."—*Rick Cerone, Former Major League Baseball Player*

PLAY BALL

DON'T LET INJURIES SIDELINE YOU THIS SEASON

DR. CHRISTOPHER AHMAD
JOHN GALLUCCI JR., MS, ATC, PT, DPT

Post Hill
PRESS

A POST HILL PRESS BOOK
ISBN: 978-1-68261-600-0
ISBN (eBook): 978-1-68261-601-7

Play Ball:
Don't Let Injuries Sideline You This Season
© 2018 by Dr. Christopher Ahmad and John Gallucci Jr., MS, ATC, PT, DPT
All Rights Reserved

Cover art by Christian Bentulan

Post Hill Press
New York • Nashville
posthillpress.com

Published in the United States of America

Dr. Christopher Ahmad's Dedication

This book is for everyone who's involved in baseball with hope that it helps better the understanding of baseball injuries and serves to reduce these injuries.

John Gallucci has been an amazing colleague on and off the field.

My brother Greg has been my deepest source of inspiration.

My parents Shafi and Judy have been a guiding light for me for my entire life.

My wife Beth and children Charlie, Sofie, and Brady encourage and challenge me every day and everything I do is for them.

John Gallucci, Jr.'s Dedication

I would like to dedicate this book to my wife, Dawn, and my children, Stephanie and Charles. Your continual support and encouragement has provided me with the motivation to chase my dreams and accomplish my goals.

Dr. Christopher Ahmad, thank you for being a wonderful colleague and friend. It has been an honor working with you throughout the last several years and I look forward to much success in the future.

I would like to extend a special thank you to the entire JAG Physical Therapy team for their support throughout the entirety of this project. Go Team JAG!

TABLE OF CONTENTS

Foreword: Why Write This Book?.. 9

Chapter 1: *Anatomy and Biomechanics of Throwing Athletes:*
The Science of a Curveball and a Broken Ligament.......... 17

Chapter 2: *Understanding the Epidemic of Elbow Baseball Injuries* ... 31

Chapter 3: *Why the Rise in Baseball Injuries?*.................................... 34

Chapter 4: *Common Overuse Injuries*... 45

Chapter 5: *Shoulder Injuries* 67

Chapter 6: *Tommy John Surgery and Other Elbow Injuries* 78

Chapter 7: *Foot and Ankle Injuries: Causes, Treatments, and*
Avoidance.. 89

Chapter 8: *Knee Injuries: How They Occur and What We Do to*
Treat Them.. 106

Chapter 9: *Hip, Thigh, and Spinal Injuries*..................................... 121

Chapter 10: *Concussions: Dangers, Symptoms, and Treatment*........... 140

Chapter 11: *Hydration and Nutrition for the Baseball Athlete*........... 150

Chapter 12: *Biomechanics and Core Development for the*
Baseball Player 163

Chapter 13: *Strength and Conditioning*... 176

Chapter 14: *Developmental Timelines: What to Expect from*
Your Athlete 197

Chapter 15: *Little Leaguer's Elbow* 211

Chapter 16: *Capitellar Osteochondritis Dissecans (OCD)* 214

Chapter 17: *Youth Elbow Injuries, Fractures, and Avulsions*.............. 218

Chapter 18: *Elbow Stress Reaction and Stress Fractures* 222

Chapter 19: *Making Tommy John Surgery History*............................. 225

Glossary **231**
About the Authors **237**

FOREWORD: WHY WRITE THIS BOOK?

Dr. Christopher Ahmad

Patients regularly ask me, "Hey, Doc, where do you sit during Yankee games? I was looking for you at last night's game." My orthopedic colleagues ask me how I find the time to write books. The answer to both questions is the same. I sit in my doctor's office inside the Gene Monahan Athletic Training Room at Yankee Stadium during games, and, rather than watch pitch after pitch, I research and write books. I have provided onsite medical care for the players and staff for eighty-one Yankee home games. Each game requires approximately six hours of my time. As the Yankees team doctor for the last nine years, I've had the time to work on book projects.

Today, while I was writing this, Nathan Eovaldi greeted me upon entering the Yankees athletic training room. Evo is recovering from the revision Tommy John surgery and repair of the forearm flexor tendon that I performed three weeks ago. I'm still wearing blue surgical scrubs from a day starting at 6:00 a.m. at the hospital and, after completing eight surgeries, I headed to the stadium. (Many people incorrectly think being the Head Team Physician for the Yankees is my full-time job.)

"How did your surgeries go?" Evo asked me with his elbow brace on. I told him I did a bunch of surgeries, one on a young, talented pitcher who needed his elbow and his knee fixed in one surgical setting. This college pitcher first developed land leg patellar tendinitis. His ability to drive towards home plate to generate throwing power was restricted by the painful patellar tendinitis. He compensated with altered throwing mechanics that added detrimental stress to his elbow. He went on to tear his elbow ulnar collateral ligament (UCL). He required Tommy John surgery and, rather than just fix his elbow ligament, I chose to fix his underlying problem and repaired his patellar tendon. He left the hospital with a brace on his left knee and one on his right elbow. Evo said, "That's a lot of surgery on a young kid. He is going to have a tough time with his rehab, I bet." I told him if we did not recognize the impact of his knee problem and correct it, it would be equivalent to changing the tires on a car with bad wheel alignment; the tires would simply break down again soon.

My office in the Yankee Stadium Athletic Training Room is off-limits to media and even to general stadium employees. This affords some privacy and solitude and, when games begin, I take advantage of it by reflecting on the events of the day. As I review the patients I operated on during that day, I'm profoundly concerned about how more and more kids are getting hurt, particularly the elbows of young pitchers. Kids experience tremendous pressure—from within themselves and from parents, friends, and coaches. I'm concerned about the abuse kids experience when pressured to play while they're in pain. I am even more concerned with kids who experience elbow or shoulder pain and who are being encouraged to participate in showcases because they fear their entire future is determined by a single great showcase performance. I see kids committing to college as early as thirteen and fourteen years of age. Recent research I've conducted also demonstrates that some young pitchers have a cavalier attitude toward injuring their ligaments. These kids will throw in spite of pain and argue that they will require reconstructive surgery at some point anyway and it might as well be now. In fact, my research shows that 50 percent of young pitchers would have surgery simply to improve their performance, even in the absence of injury.

It is estimated that 25 percent of Major League Baseball (MLB) players have now undergone Tommy John surgery. It seems every year, we lose one of the best pitchers on the Yankees roster to ulnar collateral ligament injury. In the 2016 season, it was Chase Whitley, who was a starting pitcher for the Yankees. Unfortunately, he injured his ulnar collateral ligament. He elected to go forward with Tommy John surgery and, during his recovery, he was put on waivers by the Yankees and picked up by the Tampa Bay Rays. After sixteen months of aggressive rehabilitation, he was able to pitch back in the big leagues. And, to my surprise and enjoyment, his first day back as a Tampa Bay Ray pitching in a Major League game was, in fact, at Yankee Stadium, pitching against the Yankees. After the game, I went to the visiting clubhouse to congratulate him on his six outs without giving up any runs. He said he felt great. The satisfaction in getting a high-level pitcher back to the big leagues is one of the most satisfying joys a sports medicine physician can have. However, the success of many players clouds the number of players who don't make it back.

Yankees Senior Vice President and General Manager Brian Cashman, on the Pitch Smart program, tells a story of Andrew Brackman, who was a No. 1 draft pick by the Yankees in 2007 with a known ligament tear and who, in fact, underwent Tommy John surgery soon after his contract was signed. He never made it back to being the player he was and his baseball career was cut short in the minor leagues. Media reports indicate that upon quitting baseball, he pursued basketball as a career in Europe—a sport that does not rely on a perfect UCL ligament.

Allowing kids to live their dreams is why we are committed to being the best physicians we can be in sports medicine. The chances of any given athlete making it from high school or college to the professional level is daunting. The National Federation of State High School Associations warns that fewer than 0.1 percent of kids who play sports will get a scholarship. Fifty percent of baseball injuries are from overuse, and 60 percent of these injuries could have been avoided with simple measures. The repetitive baseball motions, in combination with young age, specialization, and professionalism, fatigue muscles and cause tissue stress without allowing for recovery.

Baseball enjoys a tremendous obsession with analytics and, as I analyze my research to date, I have published over 150 articles related to baseball injuries and have given over 100 lectures to educate others on baseball-related topics such as Tommy John surgery. However, these academic works were designed to help doctors take better care of their baseball player patients and, therefore, does not speak to the issue that matters most: the players themselves, the parents, and the coaches. This book is written to get to the root of the problem through education and demystifying the true factors related to baseball injuries.

John Gallucci and I connected through injury, rehabilitation, and keeping alive the dreams of athletes. I grew up playing soccer and enjoyed four years playing at nationally ranked Columbia University. John also began his athletic training career at Columbia, which is how we met. Many of my teammates went on to play at the professional level, and John Gallucci was there to rehabilitate them from their injuries, as he became the "go-to specialist" for elite athletes. I then became the Head Team Physician for the New York City Football Club, and John and I immediately took on managing soccer player injuries and rehab and injury prevention together. Together, we identified baseball as the next area for us to enact change by demystifying baseball injuries and creating a platform for improving baseball health. This book is a reference guide for parents, players, coaches, and even grandparents to educate themselves and help reduce injuries.

Anything we write about ourselves is not to celebrate our accomplishments, but, rather, to highlight our obligation to the kids and protect them from injury. I have worked with Major League Baseball with a funding of close to one million dollars to create a national multicenter Tommy John registry through MLB-supported research that will be able to answer many questions regarding Tommy John surgery. This research initiative is the first of its kind and will support athletes of all levels.

I want to thank John Gallucci, Jr., my clinical team with whom I work every day, Head Athletic Trainer Steve Donahue, and former Head Athletic Trainer of the New York Yankees Gene Monahan, who taught me the unwritten curriculum of how to manage athletes and their parents, coaches, and teammates.

John Gallucci Jr.

As I write this book, I reflect on how many Little League and youth games I have competed in as a young athlete, along with how many I have watched from the stands as a coach, parent, and medical professional. Throughout the last several years, youth sports have experienced declines in participation, and baseball hasn't escaped this trend. Since 2007, according to data from the Sports & Industry Fitness Association (SFIA), the number of kids from six to twelve years old who play baseball has fallen from 5.44 million to 4.34 million. Although there are a number of reasons for lack of participation, we want to make sure that failure to participate due to injury isn't on the top of that list.

The goal in cowriting this book is to combine my education as an athletic trainer and physical therapist, my years of experience, and my clinical aptitude to try to keep players on the field, be they Major League Baseball players, semiprofessional players, college players, high school players, club players, or just recreational players trying to keep fit. I will give a detailed look at every joint and the common baseball injuries that affect them, and will simplify the diagnosis, mechanism, treatment, and prevention of each of these injuries. I hope this book becomes a resource for players, coaches, umpires, and parents to assist in keeping our athletes safe, healthy, and playing the sport that they love.

While I was finishing my master's degree in athletic training and my doctorate in physical therapy, I was always interested in teaching athletes about how to take care of their bodies. I have always told parents, coaches, athletes, and medical professionals, "Your body is your tool. You need to take care of your tools to accomplish your goals."

Over my twenty-two-year career, I have seen many different types of sports medicine injuries. My time with New York University, Columbia University, and the New York Knicks gave me a platform of experiences and education to prepare me for the last sixteen years of my career as a sports medicine professional. It is through my work at Columbia University that I first met Dr. Christopher Ahmad. Over the years, Dr. Ahmad and I have collaborated on countless cases and have built a great relationship with one common goal in mind: keeping our athletes healthy and ready for the game.

My background in sports medicine gave me the great opportunity for a full-time position within Major League Soccer, which began when I started doing rehabilitation on surgical cases with the MetroStars. I had the opportunity to stay with the team through many changes in management and ownership as the league grew and other teams and owners were brought in. The team later became known as the New York Red Bulls, and I became their head athletic trainer.

I used that position to educate more and more soccer enthusiasts about injuries and their prevention. Major League Soccer executives were so impressed with my knowledge and experience that they made me the league's Medical Coordinator in 2006. This position has afforded me the opportunity to work with not only our players, but also soccer medicine colleagues from around the world. Again, I was given the opportunity to work hand-in-hand with Dr. Ahmad, who currently serves as the head team physician for New York City FC, one of Major League Soccer's newest teams.

Along with my background and experience in the realm of professional sports, I also own and operate JAG Physical Therapy, a private outpatient physical therapy company with seventeen facilities in New Jersey and New York. At JAG Physical Therapy, I treat patients of all ages, shapes, and sizes, which allows me to utilize my expertise on not only the professional athlete, but on the youth athlete and weekend warrior, as well. Whether you are playing your first game as a child, or are a businessman kicking the ball around with a few friends, injuries can occur. I work hard every day to get people back to 100 percent so they can continue doing what they love to do.

Throughout years of working in collaboration with Dr. Ahmad, we have seen a recent influx in baseball injuries that required surgery followed by extensive post-operative physical therapy. Specifically, UCL (ulnar collateral ligament) injuries in athletes have resulted in a rapid rise of Tommy John surgery. Twenty-five percent of active MLB pitchers have had the procedure, which reconstructs a pitcher's torn UCL. What is immediately alarming is that more pitchers had the surgery in 2014 than in the entirety of the 1990s.

With the recent data coming out about injuries to the baseball athlete, various questions are being asked. Why are more young athletes undergoing surgery? What can athletes do to avoid injury? Is Tommy John surgery necessary for young athletes? What is the success rate of Tommy John surgery? We can go on and on with the myriad of questions that are being asked of medical professionals each and every day. The goal in writing this book is to provide extensive knowledge and insight into the most common baseball injuries to educate the community in order to help decrease the incidence of injury.

I would like to thank Dr. Ahmad for collaborating with me on this project. When you think of sports medicine, you immediately think of Dr. Christopher Ahmad and the work he has done to stay at the forefront of the injury epidemic. His commitment to his patients, research, and evolving science of medicine is unparalleled, and I consider myself honored to have my name published alongside his.

A NOTE ABOUT THIS BOOK

The overriding structure and message of this book is decidedly a joint effort between Dr. Christopher Ahmad and John Gallucci, Jr. However, they elected to apply their unique areas of expertise to specific aspects of this book and divided the chapters accordingly. This enables readers to enjoy first-person descriptions of people and circumstances each of the authors have encountered. The chapters indicate the primary author of each chapter. Readers should feel assured that both authors reviewed and contributed to the entire book.

CHAPTER 1
by Dr. Christopher Ahmad

ANATOMY AND BIOMECHANICS OF THROWING ATHLETES: THE SCIENCE OF A CURVEBALL AND A BROKEN LIGAMENT

PITCHING BIOMECHANICS

A three-inch diameter baseball weighing five ounces routinely lights up 95 mph on the radar gun when thrown by Major League pitchers. This equates to a velocity of 139 feet per second during the 60-foot, six-inch path to home plate, with a flight duration of 4/10ths of a second. I observed Aroldis Chapman, when playing as a Yankee, throw a fastball 104 mph that reached home plate in 380 milliseconds. Blink, and you don't see the pitch, but you do hear the thunderous pop of the catcher's mitt.

The pitching motion is perhaps the most complex and forceful movement in all of sports and the subject of extensive research. In fact, the pitching motion is the fastest human movement ever recorded. It breaks down to a series of synchronized component movements requiring precise coordination of close to one hundred muscles, bones, and soft tissue structures. The repetitive throwing motion challenges the strength and durability of these tissues that, unfortunately, leads to predictable injury patterns in pitchers.

Pitch velocity starts in the large mass of the lower extremities as kinetic energy that is eventually transferred to the ball like a whip snapping. The "kinetic chain" is a term used to describe the sequence of activation, mobilization, and stabilization of different body segments. The strongest and largest muscle in the body—the gluteus maximus—initiates the motion. In fact, half of the total energy and force developed in throwing is produced in the legs and the trunk, and, so, it follows that ball velocity correlates more with lower body strength than upper body strength. During wind-up, the pitcher loads his back leg in preparation for a forceful drive toward home plate. His shoulder and arm move into a position that ultimately creates a whipping action. The pitcher's straight-line acceleration toward home plate carries his entire body mass, which then abruptly decelerates when his land leg strikes the front of the mound. The tremendous momentum created during the linear drive toward home plate by the legs and trunk abruptly transfers to rotational force in the upper extremity, which has moved into a cocking position. The arm then rapidly rotates toward home plate like a whip accelerating the five-ounce ball. Arm rotation velocities as high as 7,000 degrees per second have been recorded, which is roughly the speed your car tire is rotating when driving 500 mph. This is the fastest recorded human movement.

Figure 1.1

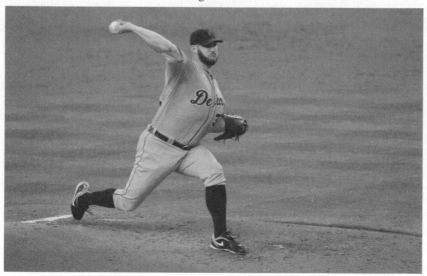

Pitching itself is mystical and even unnatural. The mechanics of pitching have been studied in the laboratory using specialized cameras and by analyzing muscle activity. The moment during a pitch that puts the shoulder and elbow at the highest risk for injury is the late cocking phase and the point where the arm is most rotated backwards as shown in Figure 1.4. When the arm reaches maximum external rotation, the energy created from driving toward home plate is converted rapidly into kinetic energy as the arm rotates toward home plate. The conversion of kinetic energy creates tremendous stress on the shoulder and the elbow. This puts the component pieces of the shoulder labrum and rotator cuff at high risk for injury. The inside part of the elbow experiences tremendous force, which finds resistance through the ulnar collateral ligament, and the back part of the elbow experiences large forces that can result in bone spur formation.

SHOULDER – INTERNAL IMPINGEMENT

The predicament of the pitcher's shoulder, at times referred to as "the thrower's paradox," describes the delicate balance between having enough mobility to foster extreme rotations while maintaining adequate stability to prevent the ball from shifting within the socket that can injure the surrounding tissues. The pitching motion has been divided into six phases. Many pitchers seek perfect mechanics, but also incorporate their own style into pitches, particularly during the wind-up and follow-through phases. Regardless of the appearance of the pitch during these phases, correct pitch mechanics are critical for effectiveness and injury prevention. Improper mechanics at any stage during this energy transfer can lead to injury and affect performance. An experienced coach educated in throwing mechanics is invaluable to the young athlete in preventing and recovering from injury by detecting and correcting subtle abnormalities. High-speed video evaluation is a useful tool to give pitchers visual feedback about their technique.

The scapula or wing blade is extremely important as it links the lower half of the body to the upper half and is a focal point of energy transference. The scapula is often underappreciated in developing pitchers. When the forces are greatest, during extreme external shoulder rotation, the cocked shoulder depends on the rotator cuff to keep the humeral head or shoulder ball centered in the socket. In addition, the labrum, which is the soft tissue lining of the socket, can be ripped away from its attachment site if the ball shifts from the center of the socket. Therefore, rotator cuff tears and labral tears are extremely common in throwing athletes.

PHASES OF PITCHING

Figure 1.2

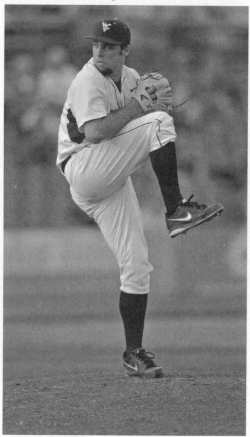

Phase (1) Wind-Up

The wind-up establishes the foundation for the remainder of the pitch, and poor wind-up mechanics can infiltrate the remaining pitch phases. The feet are positioned parallel to one another and perpendicular to the rubber on the mound as the pitcher faces the batter. A right-handed pitcher then places the right foot parallel to the rubber. As the left leg is elevated, the pitcher keeps the hips level to the ground and points them toward home plate while maintaining balance. The hips then begin driving forward toward home plate, and the right hand with the ball exits the left-hand glove.

During the wind-up phase, the pitcher should be balanced when the leading leg reaches its highest point. If the pitcher begins to fall forward prematurely as a result of poor balance, the delivery is rushed, and the velocity on the pitch will be lessened. If the hips fail to point toward home plate, the leading leg will land in an incorrect direction during subsequent pitch phases.

Figure 1.3

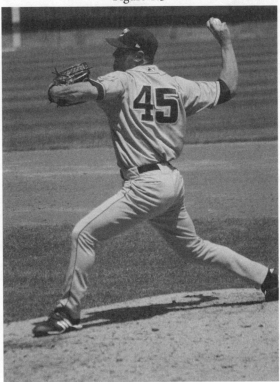

Phase (2) Early Cocking

The hand comes out of the glove while maintaining a position on top of the ball and the shoulder remains rotated inward. As the hand brings the ball back and away from the body, the hips drive toward home plate, but the pelvis does not rotate. The phase ends with the left foot landing on the mound, which decelerates the driving lower extremity and trunk.

Two common errors should be avoided in this phase: "pie throwing" and "opening up" too soon. First, if the hand is rotated under the ball instead of remaining on top, the arm rotates outward and places the shoulder joint into a vulnerable position for anterior subluxation and instability. Second, the lead foot should land pointing toward home plate. Flaws observed in inexperienced pitchers include moving the lead leg away from the body when landing on it. For example, a right-handed pitcher with poor form would place the lead left foot on the first-base side of the mound. This premature opening causes early pelvis rotation with a subsequent loss of velocity and increased shoulder strain. Movement of the high-mass lower extremity and trunk creates maximal energy in the lower body that is transferred to the upper extremity and, finally, to the ball. This requires timed and delayed upper body rotation to allow lower extremity and trunk energy to develop.

Figure 1.4

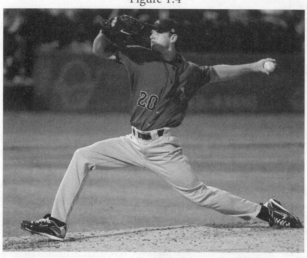

Phase (3) Late Cocking

Most injured pitchers experience pain during the late cocking phase. During this phase, at maximal external rotation (nearing 170 degrees), the arm should move away from the midline of the body 90 to 100 degrees. Decreasing external rotation at the time of foot contact may be associated with increased strain on the anterior shoulder during acceleration and ball release.

In late cocking, the left foot hits the ground pointing toward home plate, leaving the legs stretched apart. The weight of the pitcher's body is evenly distributed on both legs with the torso balanced upright between the legs. Trunk rotation is delayed as long as possible while the right arm externally rotates from approximately 45 degrees to 170 degrees.

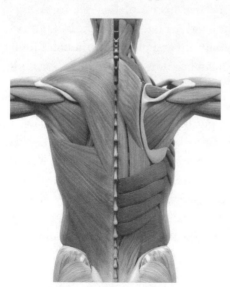

Periscapular muscular weakness may also predispose athletes to injury during the late cocking phase. The serratus anterior is significantly less active in pitchers with shoulder instability than in pitchers with normal shoulders. To compensate for diminished serratus anterior strength, the thrower might drop the elbow, thus decreasing the degree of scapular rotation and elevation needed. If this process continues, the player might compensate even further by moving the

Figure 1.5

arm behind the body. If symptoms arise, players decrease the amount of external rotation to protect against shoulder pain and arch the back to compensate for the decreased external rotation in their arm. Early recognition of muscle imbalances in the thrower can allow the surgeon to institute an early, focused physical therapy program to strengthen the affected structures and protect against the vicious cycle of compensatory throwing.

The elbow should reach its highest point in late cocking (see Figure 1.4); immature throwers often have their elbows in a suboptimal lower position.

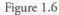

Figure 1.6

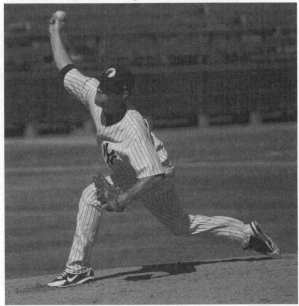

Phase (4) Acceleration

Once the arm reaches maximal outward rotation, the hand carrying the ball accelerates in a rapid arc of inward rotation. The lower extremity and trunk energy is transferred through the shoulder to the elbow and wrist as the body falls forward. Immediately prior to ball release, the arm internally rotates 80 degrees, reaching peak angular velocities near 7,000 degrees per second. Within 0.05 seconds, the ball is released with speeds exceeding 90 mph.

Pitchers who lead with the elbow, or keep their arms closer to the midline of their bodies while increasing elbow flexion to bring the ball closer to the shoulder, might also relieve a painful shoulder during the acceleration phase. Although this maladaptive position decreases the load on the shoulder, it increases the load on the medial elbow, encouraging injury. If the thrower opens up too quickly, positioning the elbow behind the plane of the scapula, the shoulder joint hyperangulates, resulting in more pronounced internal impingement.

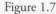

Figure 1.7

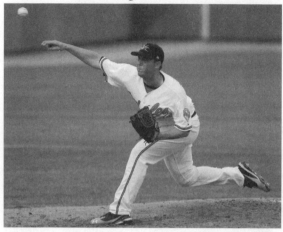

Phase (5) Deceleration

After ball release, the right hip rises up and over the left leg. The right foot lifts off the mound and the body performs a controlled fall forward. In this phase, the rotator cuff muscles contract to dissipate the kinetic energy that was not transferred to the ball. The shoulder forces, which are absorbed by the shoulder capsule and posterior rotator cuff, can reach 1 to 1.5 times body weight at this time.

Figure 1.8

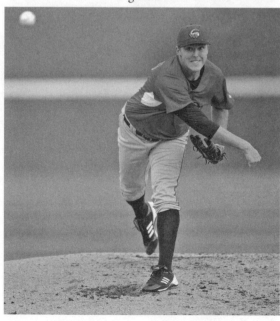

Phase (6) Follow-through

The arm continues to descend, and the right leg lands on the ground in a controlled fashion. The arm decelerates as the rotator muscles contract, and, as the arm moves toward the midline of the body, the posterior capsule tenses. During the follow-through, the shoulder should rotate inward and move horizontally across the body. If instead the arm finishes facing home plate, the shoulder will stress excessively.

Injury patterns in the shoulder and elbow can occur from injuries anywhere in the kinetic chain. The kinetic chain mechanism to generate ball velocity is extremely sensitive to alteration. For example, hamstring tightness, hip rotation deficits, or spine inflexibility can all result in even minute kinetic chain alterations that then increase stress on the shoulder and elbow, leading to injury. In fact, studies show that rotator cuff or labral tears in the shoulder are very often associated with a problem somewhere else in the athlete's body or throwing motion. Therefore, the entire kinetic chain must be evaluated in any injured throwing athlete and should be assessed prior to play so it can be corrected to reduce further injury.

ANATOMY – WHAT'S REALLY GOING ON DURING A PITCH?

The shoulder is a ball-and-socket joint and achieves its range of motion with an inherited risk of injury. The rotator cuff muscles stabilize the ball within the socket. The socket is relatively flat, and the surrounding tissue, called the labrum, functions like a washer, deepening the socket and creating stability. It is common for throwers to develop injuries to the labrum and to the rotator cuff.

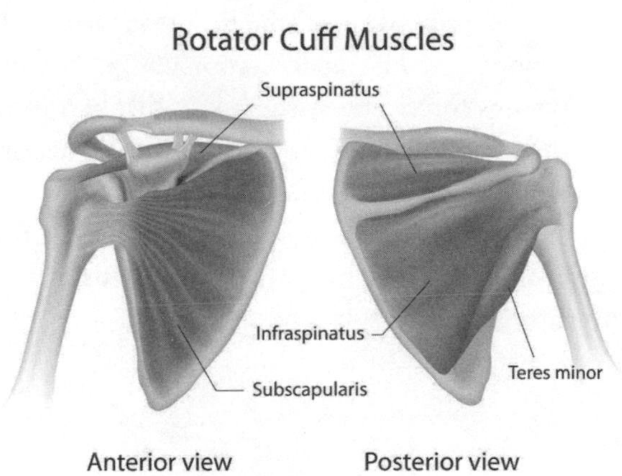

Rotator Cuff Muscles

Supraspinatus

Infraspinatus

Subscapularis

Teres minor

Anterior view   Posterior view

Figure 1.9

Ulnar Collateral Ligament

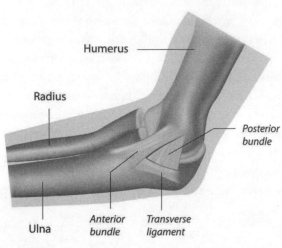

Figure 1.10

The elbow is a hinged joint that resembles a spool on one end with a perfectly matched shape on the surface of the other end. Throwing stretches, or otherwise distracts, forces on the inside of the elbow as the ball accelerates. The stretching force is counterbalanced primarily by the UCL that attaches the humerus and ulna bones like a rope. The UCL is, therefore, essential to throwing and is frequently injured. The muscles of the elbow can greatly stabilize the distracting forces and protect the UCL, which was a critical discovery in my research laboratory. The muscles can be modified through exercise, whereas the ligament cannot. Therefore, the elbow muscles are emphasized in rehabilitation and prevention programs.

The elbow also sees forces across the bones that can form bone chips and spurs that can become painful. In addition, the forearm muscles are stressed during throwing and can be further injured in the form of muscle strains. Since the forearm musculature protects the UCL, any player with a forearm muscle injury should be fully recovered prior to returning to activity to protect the UCL from injury.

BIOMECHANICS OF LIGAMENT TEARS

As the pitcher accelerates the five-ounce ball, the force on the UCL approaches 60 pounds. This is similar to five bowling balls hanging from your wrist while in the cocking position of throwing. The forearm essentially wants to detach from the body, which was how Tommy John felt when his UCL tore. The UCL is a two-inch ligament in the elbow that holds two bones together like a rope. But ligament is different from muscle and can't be strengthened through exercise as muscles can. A professional pitcher's ligament is pretty much the same as a soccer player's or a surgeon's, and there is little he can do to make it stronger.

I studied mechanical engineering at the School of Engineering and Applied Science at Columbia University. The academic work included engineering labs where we pulled materials apart to understand the strength of materials and their breaking characteristics. I was later fascinated with the vulnerability of the UCL. After testing dozens of cadaver UCLs in the lab in 2000, I was stunned to discover that the ligament breaks at 32 newton meters. This is shocking because throwing a baseball imposes a force of 50 newton meters on the UCL—this suggests that the UCL should tear with every pitch.

Why then does the ligament not break with each pitch? This question has guided my research for the last fifteen years. One hypothesis is that the muscles of the forearm and elbow, which are positioned over the top of the ligament, provide protection to the ligament. We created an experiment that simulates this muscle activity and proved our hypothesis that the muscles of the elbow have a huge effect on shielding the UCL from stress. The importance of this discovery is that forearm muscles can be strengthened even though ligaments can't. Athletic trainers, physical therapists, and others involved in baseball health now emphasize muscle development and health in baseball players. A more recent and sobering study I performed this year analyzed the effects of a forearm muscle strain, a common injury in big league pitchers. Our data indicates that 20 percent of pitchers who attempt to return to play after a forearm strain will go on to require Tommy John surgery within one year.

THE CURVEBALL CONTROVERSY – DOES IT MATTER WHAT TYPE OF PITCH IS THROWN?

Studies in the pitching laboratory examined different pitch types searching for an algorithm that could protect the throwing elbow and shoulder. In particular, the curveball has been analyzed extensively. Research tells us consistently that the biggest indicator of increased ligament stress is higher pitch velocity. The exact performance measure that scouts and coaches most seek is, possibly, the biggest risk factor! How can we possibly prevent or cure injury, then?

The hardest-throwing athletes and those who develop velocity at a young age have more stress on their UCL. The change-up or off-speed pitch, which has significantly less velocity compared to the fastball, shows the least amount of stress in the laboratory. In between are the breaking pitches between the fastball and the change-up, which includes the curveball and the slider. There are anecdotal claims that youth pitchers who throw curveballs modify their throwing mechanics and are more prone to injury. This has not been shown in the laboratory. The ideal mechanics for throwing for any given pitcher is still yet to be determined, but it is clear that mechanics do deteriorate with overuse and fatigue. We observed several positional changes in collegiate players who pitch deep into games or toward the end of a season.

WHY DOES A TEN-YEAR-OLD THROWING A CURVEBALL CAUSE SO MUCH CONCERN FOR ELBOW INJURY?

Young pitchers are often injured due to irresponsible training and by forcing competitive skills that are more suited for older players. There are currently no rules in baseball restricting the use of the curveball. USA Baseball, the governing body for amateur baseball in this country, recommends that breaking pitches (curveballs, sliders, and so forth) not be thrown until after bone maturity. These recommendations were formulated based on expert opinion.

One research study that used postgame telephone interviews of 476 youth pitchers for one season asked the questions, "Did you feel any pain in your elbow from pitching?" and, "Did you feel any pain in your shoulder from pitching?" A comparison between pitchers who reported throwing curveballs and pitchers who only threw fastballs found a 1.52 odds' increase in shoulder pain in the former group. Although this study has not been reproduced consistently, it has been postulated that youth pitchers with the highest pitch counts are likely the better pitchers on the team and, therefore, are more inclined to throw a curveball earlier in their careers, further introducing overuse as a confounding variable. Essentially, players who throw curveballs likely have additional reasons, such as overuse, as the cause of injury.

The other study supporting USA Baseball's recommendation, a retrospective review of twenty-seven pitchers who underwent ulnar collateral ligament reconstruction, reported that sixteen of twenty-four patients threw a curveball before the age of fourteen. It should be noted that this observation was not compared to a healthy age-matched control group to determine the statistical significance of this result. A more recent study attempted to mitigate the lack of a study control group. Another research study compared ninety-five pitchers who underwent arm surgery to forty-five uninjured pitchers and found no correlation of injury to the age at which the curveball was first thrown. Consequently, the evidence supporting limiting youth from using the curveball comes from flawed studies. Two studies, however, did find that throwing a change-up pitch reduced the incidence of elbow and/or shoulder pain.

The ten biomechanical studies examined the motion of pitching a curveball and have not shown that the mechanical differences increased the strain on a pitcher's shoulder or elbow. Consistent differences in arm position among the studies included: increased elevation of the shoulder, increased forearm rotation, and decreased wrist extension. Yet no increase in kinetics was observed in the shoulder or elbow. Of particular note, there is no indication that there is additional stress to the elbow potentially injuring the UCL. The current evidence does not support limiting the use of curveballs at any level of baseball. We support USA Baseball's recommendation to teach proper mechanics and learn the change-up, as this pitch may protect against arm injuries. In addition, as overuse remains the one consistent risk factor for injury, further biomechanical analysis of upper extremity strain caused by overuse will improve our understanding of the increasing incidence of baseball pitching injuries.

Despite much debate in the baseball community about the safety of the curveball, biomechanical and most epidemiological studies do not indicate an increased risk of pain and/or injury when compared to the fastball. Current recommendations to discourage throwing curveballs at a young age, while well intentioned, are based on observational data and expert opinion that have not been validated by biomechanical studies. According to the available evidence, it is possible that, with supervised attention to proper form and technique, youth pitchers may safely use the curveball without incurring increased risk of injury. Many pitching coaches now advocate throwing a curveball when a player demonstrates the ability to spin the ball on flat ground without mechanical pitching flaws.

Take winning out of the equation and place development first.

CHAPTER 2
by Dr. Christopher Ahmad

UNDERSTANDING THE EPIDEMIC
OF ELBOW BASEBALL INJURIES

Are more pitchers actually hurting their elbows, or are the sports doctors just getting better at diagnosing injuries? Are pitchers just more open about admitting their injuries, or are teams just more liberal about prescribing the surgeries?

YOUTH PARTICIPATION

Sixteen million youth baseball players exist, and it's estimated that up to 20 percent of them between the ages of nine to fifteen will seek medical attention. The estimated medical costs of these injuries is close to 1.8 billion dollars, and 50 percent of these injuries are related to overuse, meaning they are preventable, especially for the pitcher, who is the most vulnerable player on the field.

At the time of this writing, the prevalence of UCL reconstruction in professional baseball pitchers at the major league level is 25 percent, and these numbers are increasing rapidly. The biggest increase is for second-time Tommy John surgery. Even more concerning is that the seventeen- and eighteen-year-old age group is undergoing Tommy John surgery at rates that exceed all other age groups. In fact, in 2017, I published research demonstrating that Tommy John surgery is at an all-time high. It used to be that my office would be filled with college athletes and some professional athletes. Now, my clinic is filled with injured high school and middle school athletes.

In New York State, between 2002 and 2011, Tommy John surgery increased 193 percent. The first decade of the 21st century has seen a tenfold increase in UCL reconstructions in Major League Baseball, and that trend continues to climb. Mainstream national media has described this phenomenon as an epidemic of Tommy John surgery.

PROFESSIONAL-LEVEL CONSIDERATIONS

I accepted an invitation to join the MLB UCL research task force initiated by then-MLB commissioner Bud Selig because more pitchers had UCL surgery in 2014 than in the entirety of the 1990s. In Major League Baseball, from 2000 through 2011, there were approximately sixteen pitchers per year who underwent UCL reconstruction, peaking at twenty in the 2007 season. From 2012 to 2014, the number increased to thirty-six per year. Also concerning is the increasing incidence of recurrent UCL tears requiring revision UCL reconstruction. At the professional levels, the figures are even more staggering. Since the first operation forty-one years ago, just shy of one thousand known UCL surgeries have been performed on major and minor league players, the vast majority of them pitchers. Seventy percent of the procedures occurred in the past decade.

The major question and concern that has only recently been elucidated by my research team is how well athletes perform following Tommy John surgery. It was previously considered an operation with an 80 to 90 percent success rate; however, that success was based solely on an athlete's ability to get back to pitching. More recently, we've looked at pitching performance metrics and we found that 80 percent return to pitch at least one Major League game; however, only 67 percent return to their prior levels of competition. Even more discouraging was the fact that 50 percent were returned to the disabled list after the surgery because of injury to their throwing arms.

My research team reviewed 147 Major League Baseball pitchers and, for the first time, described what their outcome was with regard to the return to standard pitching metrics. We found that, although the majority of players were able to return to competition, approximately 80 percent—a large percent of players who were established Major League pitchers—were unable to return to their previous level of competition.

Return to competition is one of the most documented metrics of success after surgery. Prior studies done by my institution report the return rates are between 80 and 90 percent for simply getting back to competition. If we examine the durability of returning to sport and stratify success as "appearing in greater than ten games during a single season after surgery," only 67 percent of players were able to return to a similar level of competition postoperatively. We also note that more than 50 percent of players return to the disabled list because of injuries to the throwing arm at some point after their return from surgery.

Following Tommy John surgery, we found significant declines in performance statistics such as ERA, batting averages against, percentage of pitches thrown in the strike zone, number of innings pitched, percentage of fastballs thrown, and average fastball velocity. The study concludes that, although professional pitchers return to MLB competition after Tommy John surgery, a return to established and durable levels of competition is less guaranteed. It is currently believed that young pitchers who are still developing and improving their performance can continue to do so after Tommy John surgery, including, for example, maintaining their velocity. The surgery, however, does not in itself improve performance.

In addition, our technical capabilities advance as new statistical measures develop. For example, PITCHF/x is a tracking system that can analyze sixty variables within baseball, tracking the 660,000 pitches thrown annually. These tools help us understand the epidemiology and significance of injuries in baseball, as well as evaluating performance as more and more data is gathered.

The reality is there are more surgeries. Are there more surgeries because there are more injuries, or are there more surgeries because we're better at finding the injuries? Or, when we find them, are the doctors more willing to do surgery? Or, are patients more willing to have surgery? This isn't an epidemic in the same way the swine flu was an epidemic, but it creates tremendous concern.

CHAPTER 3
by Dr. Christopher Ahmad

WHY THE RISE IN
BASEBALL INJURIES?

How do you keep a pitcher from getting hurt?

There's only one right answer. Don't let him pitch.

Ten years ago, when I first started as the Yankees Head Team physician, high school draft picks had good-looking (meaning: normal) elbows on their MRI scans. Today, a typical eighteen-year-old high school draft pick player looks more like a thirty-year-old veteran free agent, with chronic ossification and arthritis in his elbow. I have the responsibility of evaluating the health and injury risk of potential players with the Yankees as part of their contract. This requires reviewing X-rays and MRI scans of the potential players' shoulders and elbows. Ten years ago, a high school draft pick would easily "pass" his physical. Now, high school players commonly demonstrate UCL thickening with calcification, prior Tommy John surgery, bone spurs, and undersurface rotator cuff tears and labral tears. Often, this leads to concern for future ability to play and, at times, leads to not signing the player—failing the physical.

Five years ago, when I evaluated injured players in my clinic, some professional and collegiate athletes would come to the appointment with their strength and conditioning coaches. Kids would come with their parents. Now, high school kids, and even thirteen-year-old kids, come to see me with their strength and conditioning coaches. They also have mental conditioning coaches, nutritionists, and yoga instructors at this young age. They have access to performance improvement strategies once reserved for professional athletes. Over the past few years, the pressure on young athletes to perform at higher levels has escalated radically. Playing baseball was once a fun activity for kids who could design their own rules and scoring systems in makeshift fields in the neighborhood. Now, youth baseball is a means for parents to create elite athletes through early professional training. Early specialization is now the major cause of overuse injuries in developing baseball players.

SPORT SPECIALIZATION AND EARLY PROFESSIONALISM

Overuse of the shoulder and elbow is now a problem for a player at any level or age and is rooted in overzealous specialization and early professionalism. I began researching this phenomenon five years ago, and this research now indicates that kids are specializing in baseball and, specifically, as pitchers, as early as eight years of age, which is not shocking since travel teams begin competing as early as age six. Athletes are encouraged to commit to a single sport by coaches before they fully experience alternate sports that may interest them more.

Four elements define an early specialist:
- Early starting age in a sport.
- Early involvement in a single sport instead of diversification.
- Early intense, focused training.
- Early involvement in competition.

Early specialization in a single sport is one of the strongest predictors of future injury in any sport, with such athletes 70 to 90 percent more likely to be injured when compared to children who play multiple sports. Baseball players are at specific risk for elbow and shoulder injuries. It has been my experience that young athletes who injure their shoulders and elbows have serious overuse problems related to early specialization. Surgery can also be the final consequence of injury, and pitchers who compete in leagues more than eight months a year or play on multiple teams are significantly more likely to need the surgery by the time they are in college.

Why is specialization so risky? Answer: Single sport athletes are subjected to overemphasized competition. This yields a series of ramifications such as a lack of physical and mental rest, playing year-round, playing on multiple teams, little or no periodization of activity, constant repetition of the same athletic movements, and a lack of the many athletic benefits of multisport participation. In addition to injury, early specialization causes burnout. Three out of four children quit sports because sports are no longer enjoyable or because they are injured. Specialization and early professionalism costs more parental financial support, which, in turn, creates even more pressure on children. Children may feel trapped with a singular identity completely associated with their sporting success. The pressure and stress can make them quit long before they ever achieve their athletic potential.

Several factors have influenced playing sports beyond childhood. First is intrinsic motivation—the "currency of athletic performance." Intrinsic motivation creates drive and grit that fuels playing through hard times. Second is enjoyment. Many of the stakeholders in youth sports fail to respect the need for fun. Third is autonomy: Young athletes thrive when they have ownership over their sports experience. Parents and coaches should support their child's drive and efforts to achieve their goals and dreams.

Athletes motivated extrinsically by championships, fame, and social identity tied to athletic success have been shown to burn out at a much higher rate than athletes who participate for enjoyment. They are also more likely to protect that identity through cheating and other maladaptive behaviors designed to continue successful outcomes.

An algorithm has been studied with success that recommends that at age twelve, 80 percent of kids' time should be spent in deliberate play and in sports *other than* the chosen sport. Age thirteen–fifteen: a 50/50 split between a chosen sport and other athletic pursuits. Age sixteen-plus: Even when specialization becomes very important, 20 percent of training time should still be in the nonspecialized sport and deliberate play.

HOW TO GET TO 10,000 HOURS WITHOUT SPECIALIZING

Why the push for specialization? I consider myself a sports medicine specialist. After all, "skill," by definition, is the ability to improve with repeated practice in that activity, and I have been practicing for fifteen years. A 2013 American Medical Society for Sports Medicine survey found that 88 percent of college athletes surveyed participated in more than one sport as a child. Abraham Lincoln once said, "Give me six hours to chop down a tree and I will spend the first four sharpening the axe."

Playing multiple sports sharpens the axe in this metaphor. Free play and multisport play promotes the development of better all-around athleticism. As children play less and practice more (often in a single sport) using sport-specific muscles and movements, experts in many sports have noticed a decline in the agility, balance, and coordination skills of young athletes as compared to decades ago. Even more important, play stimulates brain development. It hastens the growth of emotion, attention, and behavior control. Free play inspires thinking and adaptation, creative problem solving, and conflict resolution. It allows children to build their own games, define their own rules, and develop the cognitive skills that are needed not only for athletics, but also in every other aspect of life.

Multiple sport participation leads to better overall motor and athletic development, longer playing careers, increased ability to transfer sports skills to other sports, increased motivation, ownership of the sports experience, and confidence. Multisport participation at the youngest ages yields better decision creativity. Athletes able to "read the game" in one sport are more apt to be equally adept in another, similar sport, and thus, their ability transfers from one sport to another. Early diversification reduces the risk of burnout and dropout and the risk of your athlete developing maladaptive psychological behaviors, such as identifying their worth with their sport performance. What if your child only liked one sport, like a picky eater who only likes pasta? We would not let our children avoid other food groups simply because they prefer a single food.

Another concern is being too involved with too many sports. Even well-intentioned parents, in trying to ensure their child is not a single-sport specialist, can accidently manufacture a multisport specialist, with swimming at 6:00 a.m., soccer at 4:00 p.m., and basketball at 7:00 p.m. I think one organized sport per season, especially for kids ten and under, is entirely appropriate.

Statistics puts pursuits into perspective. About 10 percent of elite ten-year-old athletes are still elite at eighteen, and only 8 percent of Nobel Prize champions were child prodigies. In fact, the only thing that early success guarantees is…early success. Your child's high-level sports career will likely only last 25 percent of his or her life. On the other hand, the lessons they learn, and their relationship with you, their parent, must last a lifetime.

Your knowledge and wisdom as an adult can guide your child down a path that not only gives them a great chance at becoming an elite performer, but, more importantly, an elite human being.

THE ISSUES WITH SHOWCASES

The next risk factor is showcases. They are conducted with lots of variation, but consistent with kids intending to impress a high school coach or college scout. The timing of showcases may be awkward, such as the middle of the winter, where the athlete is out of shape or coming off a minor injury. The showcases require hard throwing, often with inadequate warm-up. It is not just pitchers. I had a patient come to me with an elbow UCL tear following a showcase as a catcher. He was asked to throw fifty balls as hard as he could to second base without any warm-up. He felt a pop on throw number twenty-two.

THE CHALLENGE OF PRECOCIOUS VELOCITY

We know velocity has a direct mathematical relationship with stress on the ulnar collateral ligament, which implies that a pitcher who throws 99 mph has an increased risk of tearing his ligament compared to a pitcher who throws 92 mph. We also know the average Major League fastball was 90.8 mph in 2008. In 2013, it had reached 92 mph, and eight pitchers hit triple digits. Major League pitchers who average 93 mph on their fastballs are twice as likely to end up on the disabled list the next season as pitchers whose fastball is below 90 mph. Pitchers are throwing harder than ever and, on a year-round basis, at a younger age. More pitchers can throw a baseball at 95 mph or higher than ever before in our history. The 100 mph barrier is becoming less of a barrier. The faster you throw the ball, the more chance you'll be an elite pitcher, but at the price of injury.

I had a thirteen-year-old in the office, and his dad had a notebook with his radar gun data over the last few months leading up to his injury. The radar gun emphasized over-effortful throwing and caused a decrease in learning how to pitch to create outs. Pitchers are also throwing harder now at all levels of baseball than in years past—yet another source of stress on an unrested arm. Precocious velocity tends to increase the opportunities for that player to pitch, year-round, on multiple teams, showcases, etc. Increased velocity is compounded by overuse and can have profound risk.

OVERUSE DUE TO YEAR-ROUND PARTICIPATION AND MULTIPLE TEAMS

Those pitchers who play baseball year-round without a winter rest period often play for more than one team at once. Inning limits are neglected. Pitching past the point of fatigue is a major cause of injury. Rest cures the fatigue. But year-round pitching, at a young age, simply isn't allowing younger pitchers to rest and recover.

It's pitch counts: We live in an age when pitch counts appear on a corner of our TV screens, updated after every pitch. So, clearly, they must be a big deal. But are they as big a deal as we make them out to be? Now that 120 pitches or so have become pretty much the absolute max, does it still make sense to blame high pitch counts for an uptick in Tommy John surgery? The best available current scientific evidence suggests that pitch counts, overall yearly pitching load, pitching for more than one team, and pitching through fatigue or weakness are the most significant, reproducible risk factors. Fatigue that leads to, or accentuates, poor mechanics leaves the UCL unprotected during the throwing motion and subjects the ligament to forces that can cause it to tear. The guidelines offered by Little League baseball and the recently developed MLB website Pitchsmart.com focus on modifying these risk factors, as well as others—such as type of pitch, which has less support as a risk factor—in an effort to match the science with injury prevention strategies.

BAD MECHANICS AND PITCH TYPE

Pitch type, especially the slider and curveball, has been implicated in youth injuries. However, many have tried to experimentally prove that the curveball, slider, split finger, or sinker increased stress to the elbow UCL, but no study to date has done so. More players of every age group are throwing curveballs and sliders, despite people in baseball circles stressing the importance of not throwing breaking balls too early. A general rule for the appropriate time for a young pitcher to begin throwing a curveball is when they have mastered the art of pitching mechanics.

Poor biomechanics have been implicated as one of the major risk factors that cause UCL injuries. There is little doubt that certain biomechanical flaws such as "dropping the elbow," the inverted "W" wind-up, and opening up the front side too soon increase the stress and torque on the UCL. Once again, no study has shown a direct relationship to these mechanics to injury. Despite lack of experimental evidence, these factors should be examined closely and mitigated whenever possible in young athletes. The goal of ongoing research is to better understand what factors or combination of factors contribute to injury at all levels of play. Finally, every pitcher has a slightly different throwing motion, but a widely held convention for avoiding injury is to develop a smooth, repeatable motion that uses all parts of the body in a coordinated sequence of transferrable kinetic energy.

MISPERCEPTIONS ABOUT TREATMENTS

"I will need the surgery at some point anyway, and I should get it now and over with to avoid the inconvenience later," has been said by both kids and their parents in my office. Some throw through all the alarms of an impending UCL tear with pain, fatigue, and so forth, with a cavalier attitude because they believe if they blow out their ligament, they can simply get it fixed and be better than they were before surgery. It's almost a purposeful attempt to tear their UCL so they can then get it fixed.

I was concerned that some patients want to have surgery even though their MRI looks normal and their pain is minimal. The underlying complaint was poor performance or not making a team. I decided to do a survey study asking high school pitchers, college baseball players, parents, and coaches about their attitudes toward elbow injury and surgery. I discovered shocking misperceptions. Sam Peltzman, a prominent economist, argued forty years ago that national safety regulations involving seat belt laws failed to reduce automobile deaths because people drove more recklessly when they felt safe. This became known as "The Peltzman Effect." The public believes the Tommy John procedure is far safer, more effective, and easier to return from than it really is, leading to reckless behavior. The Peltzman Effect has been observed in mountain climbing, bicycling, and skydiving.

I recently performed Tommy John surgery on an extremely competitive Yankees player. He was nearing his return to full competition at the start of spring training. I saw him at the Tampa facility in February and, while performing his preseason physical examination, I noticed he had a new tattoo on his throwing arm. Within an accurately stitched baseball, an insignia boldly read "100 mph." He was currently throwing 98 miles per hour, and the ink on his arm was a way of challenging himself to another two miles an hour.

I researched the actual performance of professional baseball players who have Tommy John surgery and found that, although 80 percent of big league pitchers who have the surgery throw again in the majors, only 67 percent of them appear in ten games or more in a single season. In addition, performance declined, as did velocity, after the surgery. Until I performed this study, general managers, coaches, agents, and players thought the surgery was automatic and that one would throw harder after the operation. The reality is that, with successful Tommy John surgery, players will develop or decline according to the many other factors that contribute to their performance.

We surveyed players, coaches, and parents and found shocking perceptions. Thirty percent of coaches, 37 percent of parents, 51 percent of high school athletes, and 26 percent of collegiate athletes believed surgery should be performed on players *without* elbow injury to enhance performance. Thirty-one percent of coaches, 28 percent of players, and 25 percent of parents did not believe the number of pitches thrown to be a risk factor, and 38 percent of coaches, 29 percent of players, and 25 percent of parents did not relate pitch type (curveballs) with risk of injury. Many players (28 percent) and coaches (20 percent) felt that performance would be enhanced over pre-injury level. In addition, our study found that a significant percentage of the public felt that Tommy John surgery could improve pitching speed, control, and overall performance over pre-injury levels. The most optimistic groups were youth and adolescent players.

Factors that drive the public misperceptions of UCL injury and surgery are now available to our youth athletes and families in the form of print, radio, television, and the Internet. Watch any Major League baseball game and a player recovering from Tommy John surgery will be highlighted with applause at the great recovery. What is not mentioned are those who did not make it back.

It is generally believed that professional pitchers serve as role models for our young athletes. Kids rank famous athletes among the most admired people in their lives, second only to their parents. It is possible that the media projection of these popular athletes performing well after surgery may explain the misperceptions of young athletes and their families regarding UCL surgery. In addition, media portrayal of pitchers may have a selection bias for successful pitchers following surgery since they still perform, as opposed to less successful procedures in those athletes who no longer perform. Players who have undergone surgery and do not get back to Major League baseball do not tend to get media attention. Therefore, professional players who have undergone Tommy John surgery and have become role models may explain why young athletes aspire to having Tommy John surgery. Possibly, the most important finding in this study was the misperception, especially in high school athletes, that surgery should be performed in the absence of injury to increase performance.

We subsequently studied media that reports on baseball games with the belief that media exerts a powerful influence on public opinion of the injury and surgery. A total of 516 members of the media with a mean age of 43.6 years completed the survey. Forty-five percent did not know if an athlete needed an elbow injury as a prerequisite for UCL reconstruction and 25 percent believed the primary indication was performance enhancement. Fifty-one percent believed return would occur in twelve or fewer months.

OVERUSE INJURIES

Fewer than half believed the use of pitch counts to be important in the prevention of UCL injury, and one-third felt that throwing injuries were *not* preventable in adolescent baseball. Common misconceptions exist regarding UCL reconstruction within the professional baseball media. Efforts for physicians to educate the media on the risks of overuse throwing injuries with emphasis on accurate indications, outcomes, and recovery of Tommy John surgery are encouraged.

CHANGING INDICATIONS FOR SURGERY

Shoulder injuries used to be the top reason for lost time in professional baseball and accounted for more than twice as many DL (Disabled List) days per year as elbow issues. Now, elbow DL time has taken over as number one and shoulder time is down. One possible reason is that pitchers are opting for Tommy John surgery at the first sign of ligament trouble, but avoid shoulder surgery because of dismal results. When a pitcher with a partial ligament tear has Tommy John, he feels, with reasonable assurance, that he'll be back in a year or so. If he opts for rest and rehab, on the other hand, his future is shrouded in mystery.

I recently operated on a pitcher with a shoulder labral tear. As part of standard protocol prior to surgery, the patient is required to sign his operative extremity. This indicates which shoulder will be operated on and is a proven systematic approach that eliminates operating accidentally on the opposite extremity. This eighteen-year-old high schooler signed his dominant throwing shoulder with his initials. Writing backwards using his non-dominant arm, he was able to scribble "95 mph please."

In recent years, a change in culture around the success of surgery has taken place. In the past, doctors recommended surgery after the ligament had been mostly or completely torn. Now, surgery to repair partial tears has become more common, a function of the surgery's success rate—defined as the chances of returning to the same level of competition or above. Professional players would often opt for earlier surgery to avoid the downside of a trial of non-operative treatment that fails, with a cost burden of three months. Surgery made more sense for these individuals. Now, college players wish to have surgery, concerned that their draft status may change if they are discovered to have missed time with elbow issues. Finally, high school kids do everything they can to preserve their junior year for the best college recruiting. If they get injured as a sophomore and surgery will get them ready in time for junior year, they usually go for the surgery. I used to spend considerable time with patients discussing the actual surgical techniques. Now, I discuss the calendar and when the earliest return possible will be. Patients already understand the surgical technique. (I may be partially responsible as I have a video demonstrating the surgical technique on YouTube.)

REVISION SURGERY

In the dozen seasons from 2000 to 2011, data from Baseballheatmaps.com indicates an average of 15.8 Major League pitchers per year had Tommy John surgery. In 2012, that number spiked to 36. From 2000 to 2013, the average number of Tommy John surgeries performed before Opening Day was only two per year. This season, there were seven—followed by four more just in the first nine days of the season. From the sixteen-year span from 1996 through 2011, the total number of pitchers who needed to repeat Tommy John came to eighteen. From 2012 to 2014, we've seen fourteen players undergo revision surgery.

The reasons for needing a second surgery are hard to understand. Is this about pitchers with flawed mechanics who come back to the same flawed mechanics? Or is it possible Tommy John surgery itself isn't the fail-safe cure it's thought to be?

CHAPTER 4
by John Gallucci, Jr.

COMMON OVERUSE INJURIES

In this chapter, we will discuss overuse injuries in baseball, but, before we continue, it is important to understand the difference between an acute injury and an overuse injury.

Acute injuries are typically the result of a single, traumatic event, such as a collision or fall, and include fractures, sprains, and dislocations. If you "hear a pop" or "feel a snap," you have likely suffered an acute injury. Overuse injuries are much subtler and their cause often cannot be traced to a specific moment. They happen over time and are the result of repetitive microtrauma to the bones, tendons, and joints.

When we exercise, bones, muscles, tendons, and ligaments get stronger as they are broken down during activity and then built back up during recovery. But if the rebuilding tissue can't keep up with the tissue breaking down, injury occurs.

As we all know, baseball is a sport that includes a lot of repetitive movements, such as running, hitting, and throwing. The specific forces placed on a baseball athlete often lead to chronic, overuse injuries. The following discusses some of these commonly seen lower extremity injuries.

ACHILLES TENDINITIS

When we're talking about any tendinitis, we're discussing a swollen or inflamed tendon. During this process, damaged tissue cells release chemicals that cause blood vessels to leak fluid into the tissue, causing swelling.

The single structure known as the Achilles tendon takes the two calf muscles—the gastrocnemius and soleus—and combines them into the tendon, connecting at the back of the heel, or calcaneus.

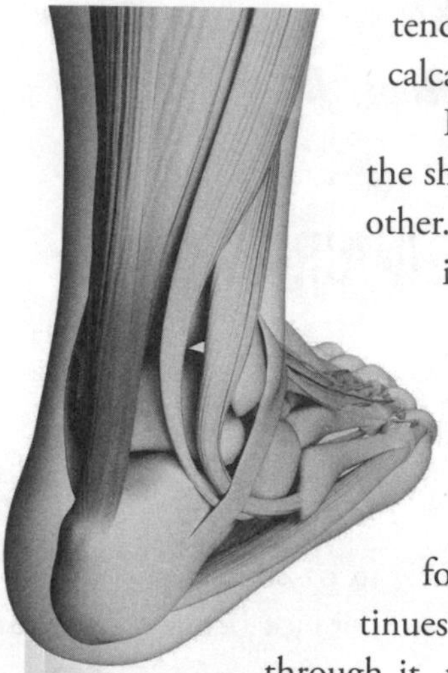

In normal, healthy tissue, the tendon and the sheath slide and glide naturally with one another. Due to repetitive actions, or even a change in intensity, the fluid released by the inflammatory response essentially takes up space within the tendon sheath, which increases the amount of friction between the tendon and the sheath. Typically, an athlete will feel some pain or discomfort when this occurs, and if he or she continues to stress the area by attempting to play through it, the inflammation will increase, leading to even less space within the tendon sheath.

Figure 4.1

Stages of Tendinitis

It is important to note the potential progression with continued use. The building effect of degenerative inflammation will damage the tissue and lead to worsening degrees of tendinitis. All types of tendinitis can vary in severity from Stage I to Stage IV.

Stage I: Pain after activity. Normal function. No gait changes; normal walking and running.

Stage II: Pain during and after activity. Athlete can still participate because warming up increases circulation and masks pain. The athlete may feel good for a short period, but there is no tendon healing.

Stage III: Prolonged pain during and after activity. Antalgic, or shortened, gait. The athlete cannot perform any activity at a satisfactory level.

Stage IV: Actual tearing of tendon, with the possibility of surgical intervention.

Achilles Tendinitis – Signs and Symptoms

Baseball players will typically complain about tightness or pain in the Achilles area in the mornings, when first getting out of bed and putting their feet on the floor. Walking loosens this up, but stationary periods lead to tightness and pain.

Athletes, as they continue to play, will also start to feel severe pain along the Achilles tendon, which, if not treated appropriately, can lead to a tear, which is a very serious injury requiring surgery and up to a year of rehabilitation. Simple tendinitis is much easier to fix, so it is important to tend to it as quickly as possible.

The area around the Achilles tendon may also visibly swell, increasing throughout the day or during activity.

How to Prevent Achilles Tendinitis

There are simple ways to prevent the onset of Achilles tendinitis as long as the baseball player adheres to a true progression of training. Simply speaking, you cannot do too much too quickly. A gradual progression from low to high intensity and frequency as certain plateaus are achieved allows proper physiological adaptations to occur at a more natural rate.

The human body is amazing and can adapt to almost any environment imaginable. Through training, we are essentially molding our bodies into the perfect tool to succeed at our sport. Close your eyes and picture Olympic weightlifters. Now, imagine all the strength training and hours spent perfecting their technique to mold their bodies into the ultimate lifting machine. Through their specific training regimen, their bodies have adapted to the external stimuli of moving heavy weight.

Of course, none of this happens overnight. Regardless of what sport we play, we must put in the training and practice hours necessary to improve our acumen for that given skill set. By gradually increasing our loads and intensity, we allow our bodies to recover and adapt at a more natural rate. We can now move on to more physically demanding activities as we build upon our foundation, striving to be the ultimate baseball player.

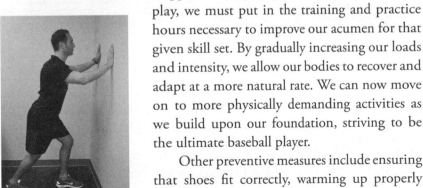

Other preventive measures include ensuring that shoes fit correctly, warming up properly before activity, and maintaining flexibility through various stretching techniques.

Figure 4.2

Also, baseball athletes should try not to change surfaces continually throughout their training regimen, meaning they should not switch between playing on concrete and playing on turf or grass frequently.

Treatment of Achilles Tendinitis

Achilles tendinitis responds very well to treatment. Central to proper treatment of tendinitis is identifying the cause of the problem, which might include:

- Change of intensity.
- A muscle not properly warmed up or stretched prior to activity.
- Training surface changes (hard and soft).
- Running too hard or too much.
- Continual, repetitive jumping and cutting.
- Changing shoes, ill-fitting shoes, or shoes that are not supportive.

By limiting or removing the cause, we can slow or reverse the inflammatory response and cure the tendinitis.

Before treating baseball athletes, it is important to recognize the way they are walking. Is there a noticeable limp? Do they favor one side over the other? Are they having difficulty decelerating, accelerating, jumping, or planting?

If the answer to any of those questions is "Yes," then the tendon likely has some level of inflammation that needs to be eliminated. The best way to accomplish this is with the RICE protocol: Rest, Ice, Compression, and Elevation.

Figure 4.3

RICE PROTOCOL	
Rest	Remove the stress. This means take a break from, change, or altogether stop any activity that increases pain or soreness.
Ice*	Three to four times per day, fifteen minutes per session, remembering not to leave on too long to avoid potential damage to the skin.

Compression	Wrap the injured area with an elastic bandage to aid in limiting inflammation.
Elevation	Use pillows to elevate the injured area while sitting or lying down. Gravity will help pull the inflammation back toward the core of the body.

*A note about icing: With soft tissue injuries, it is often more beneficial to administer an ice massage rather than to simply lay a bag of ice or frozen peas over the injured area. Freeze water in a Dixie cup, peel away the excess paper, and use the cup to massage the area. The massaging action will decrease the inflammation and pain in the area at a more efficient rate.

If pain is severe, it is advisable at this point to see a doctor for an evaluation and assessment of the direction of care. While Achilles tendinitis does not usually require surgical intervention, it can benefit from immobilization in a boot or cast to limit motion of the foot and ankle. If proper attention is paid to the injury in its early stages, it can be handled before it progresses to an aggressive stage.

If the Achilles tendinitis is only causing soreness and pain, and is not affecting the athlete's gait or performance, I recommend:

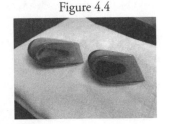

Figure 4.4

- Heel lifts bilaterally (in both shoes)
- A good warm-up and stretching
- Practice modification

As the inflammation surrounding the tendon decreases, the pain will go away! As the player starts to feel less pain and tightness in the area, based on increased flexibility and the treatment suggested, there should be a modified progression for a return to play.

With Achilles tendinitis, athletes often have great success if they return to training at 50 percent of their normal level of activity, or simply cut the athlete's workload in half—e.g., if the team is doing ten sprints, do only five. If successful, the workload builds gradually up to 75 percent, 80 percent, and, eventually, 100 percent. If the tendinitis becomes more exaggerated, the athlete should seek appropriate medical care in the form of a good physical therapist or athletic trainer.

In the clinic, we use different modalities and devices to increase circulation to the tendon, which decreases swelling and inflammation within the tendon.

The sports medicine professional then progresses with different massage and stretching techniques. When adequate time has been allowed for healing, a progression of therapeutic exercise will assist in safely returning the athlete's strength and coordination.

Once a solid foundation is laid, the athlete may progress to functional, sport-specific exercises, including running, jumping, backpedaling, and side-shuffling. As the foundation increases, more general baseball skills may be introduced. Eventually, the athlete may return to on-field activities and progress to a full return to practice.

Too many times in my career, I have seen athletes with Achilles tendinitis return to play too quickly. While an adequate course of treatment could effectively eliminate the injury, athletes are, instead, plagued by the injury throughout the season, and, often, throughout their career.

SEVER'S DISEASE

Sever's disease, or calcaneal apophysitis, is a painful bone disorder resulting from inflammation in the calcaneal epiphyseal plate, or growth plate, in the heel. A growth plate is an area of growing tissue at the end of a developing bone. Over time, cartilage cells change into bone cells, and the growth plates expand and join together, which is how bones grow.

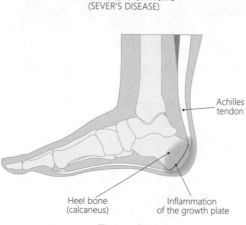

CALCANEAL APOPHYSITIS
(SEVER'S DISEASE)

Achilles tendon

Heel bone
(calcaneus)

Inflammation
of the growth plate

Figure 4.5

The calcaneal epiphyseal plate is the growth center of the heel bone where the Achilles tendon attaches at the heel. Sever's disease is a common cause of heel pain in growing kids, especially those who are very active. This condition typically arises during growth spurts in the adolescent years, between the ages of ten to fifteen for boys, and eight and thirteen for girls. During these years, adolescents experience rapid growth with immature bone transforming into fully matured bone. Sever's disease rarely occurs in older teenagers because the growth plate in the heel typically hardens by age fifteen.

Mechanism of Injury

During an adolescent's growth spurt, the heel bone can grow faster than the leg muscles and tendons around it. This causes the muscles and tendons, especially the Achilles tendon or heel cord, to become very tight and to pull directly on the growth plate in the calcaneus, or heel bone. This increase in stress and tension, which is exacerbated with activity, causes irritation at the heel. Over time, repeated stress can damage the growth plate, causing the swelling, tenderness and pain of Sever's disease.

Though Sever's disease can occur in any growing child, certain conditions, such as pes planus or flat feet, pes cavus or high arches, short leg syndrome (where one leg is shorter than the other), and childhood obesity, may increase the chances of its development.

Signs and Symptoms of Sever's Disease

The symptoms of Sever's disease are seen most often in the running athlete. Complaints most often include heel pain, tightness, swelling, and sometimes bruising. The pain will increase with running and jumping activities, and it may be exacerbated by a tight shoe.

Treatment of Sever's Disease

Identified early on, Sever's disease treatment can succeed and limits long-term difficulties that might arise. Take note of when an athlete begins to complain of heel pain so a doctor or physical therapist can assess how the symptoms are progressing.

The initial goal in treating Sever's disease is pain relief by decreasing inflammation. The best way to accomplish this is with the RICE protocol: Rest, Ice, Compression, and Elevation. (See Figure 4.3)

Figure 4.6

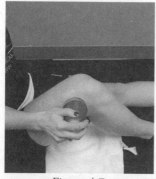

Icing at the heel is best done with an ice cup for approximately fifteen minutes, four times per day. Once the initial inflammatory response subsides, a flexibility program can begin to limit the tension being placed on the growth plate of the Achilles tendon. The goal is to increase the elasticity of the calf muscles and associated tendons that insert at the calcaneus.

Figure 4.7

Figure 4.8

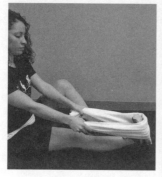
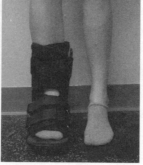

No treatment can change the course of a child's growth spurt, nor can we determine when growth spurts begin and how long they last. Should symptoms arise, they must be treated appropriately with rest and modified activity. Athletes often have to sit out for a time to allow the pain and swelling to subside. In severe cases, doctors may even choose to immobilize the foot in a cast or boot to allow healing. Once the athlete can walk without pain, a protocol to improve the strength and flexibility of the

Figure 4.9

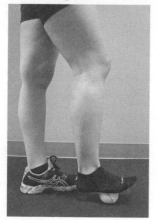

foot and heel cord are important for a successful outcome.

Remember, do not neglect the foot! Elasticity within the plantar fascia, or tissue under the foot, can also curb the symptoms of Sever's disease by dispersing the ground reaction forces experienced at the heel and above. Simple stretching is beneficial; deep-tissue massage is even better and can be done by rolling the foot on a firm ball to break up any adhesions. This same method can and should be done at the calf muscle belly.

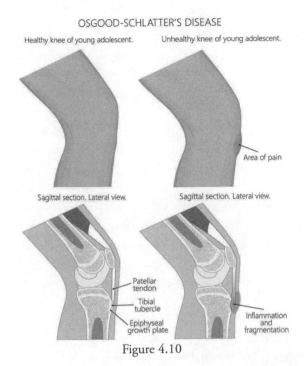

Figure 4.10

OSGOOD-SCHLATTER DISEASE

Osgood-Schlatter disease is very similar to Sever's disease, but occurs at the knee joint rather than the heel. Specifically, pain and inflammation occur at the proximal tibia where the quadriceps tendon inserts into the bone, at the bony protuberance below the kneecap. This protuberance is more prominent in some individuals and is often the result of the same force reaction that defines Sever's disease. In general, a tight quadriceps tendon pulls on the growth plate during running and jumping. When combined with rapid growth spurts in adolescent athletes, Osgood-Schlatter disease can result. Most often, it only affects one knee, and is more prevalent in boys than girls. It is very common, occurring in about 20 percent of the population, or in one of every five youth athletes.

Signs and Symptoms of Osgood-Schlatter Disease

Swelling and inflammation exist directly at the site of trauma, often with point tenderness. A visible, painful bump may develop just below the knee joint at the proximal tibia. The muscles surrounding the knee, including the hamstring and quadriceps, may be tight. Adults who experienced Osgood-Schlatter as adolescents may still have a visibly enlarged bony protuberance. This symptom can remain, and must be managed throughout an athlete's career.

Treatment of Osgood-Schlatter Disease

Symptoms of Osgood-Schlatter disease can be acutely exacerbated with activity, so there needs to be a period of RICE to reduce pain and swelling at the knee. Once inflammation is controlled, a program to increase elasticity in the surrounding musculature can begin. A good quadriceps strengthening protocol should be included, beginning with muscle-setting exercises, such as quad sets, and advancing to include closed kinetic chain (CKC) exercises. Avoiding open kinetic chain (OKC) activities will also help with this injury, since these exercises often increase symptoms. Nonsteroidal anti-inflammatory drugs, or NSAIDs, may be warranted, depending on the severity of pain and level of dysfunction.

As the athlete's pain decreases and elasticity increases, he or she can gradually return to play. Once again, while we cannot change the growth pattern of the child, we can limit symptoms of Osgood-Schlatter disease by removing activities that irritate the area. If the athlete feels good enough for batting practice, but running bases exacerbates pain, coaches need to make accommodations within the training protocol. The goal is to keep the athlete on the field, not sitting on the sideline. It is important for parents, athletes, and coaches to work together to properly manage the signs and symptoms of Osgood-Schlatter disease, and to keep the athlete under the care of a physical therapist or athletic trainer.

PATELLOFEMORAL PAIN SYNDROME

Patellofemoral pain syndrome is an overuse injury seen in youth athletes caused by friction on the cartilage under the patella, or kneecap. This causes a softening, roughening, or general degeneration of the cartilage under the kneecap known as chondromalacia.

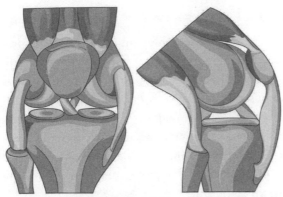

Figure 4.11

How Injury Occurs

Typically, the patella tracks in a straight line in the trochlear groove at the center of the thighbone, and pressure is spread over the widest possible area. If the patella is tilted or slides outside of this groove, pressure is uneven and can irritate the cartilage under it. Improper tracking of the kneecap can be caused by a variety of preexisting conditions, including flat feet, knock-knees, or weakness of the hip and thigh muscles.

Repeated subluxation, or partial dislocation, of the patella or trauma to the back side of the patella (the side that articulates with the trochlear groove of the femur) also causes rubbing or grinding of cartilage behind the kneecap, which has degenerative effects over time.

Signs and Symptoms of Patellofemoral Pain Syndrome

The improper mechanics of the kneecap in patellofemoral pain syndrome causes an inflammatory response, resulting in pain behind the kneecap and compensatory changes in the gait pattern. Pain may be aggravated by activity and by long periods of sitting with the knees in a moderately bent position. This is known as the "theater" or "movie-goer's" sign of patellofemoral pain syndrome. The athlete may also complain of tightness or a feeling of fullness at the front of the knee. Patellofemoral pain syndrome does not always cause crippling pain, but it can lead to debilitating degenerative changes over time.

<u>Treating Patellofemoral Pain Syndrome</u>

Patellofemoral pain syndrome is something most players can deal with and will attempt to play through. However, if not properly managed, patellofemoral pain syndrome can progress into a more severe injury that requires surgical intervention, such as a fissuring or fracturing of the patella.

Initially, a RICE protocol is essential to limit the inflammation caused by patellofemoral pain syndrome. A physician may elect to prescribe anti-inflammatory drugs, or NSAIDs. Beyond immediate treatment to manage pain and inflammation, it is essential to change the biomechanics of the knee to correct the cause of this syndrome.

The vastus medialis obliquus (VMO), which is the quadriceps muscle on the inside of the thigh, needs to fire in the proper sequence and to be sufficiently strong so it pulls the kneecap in the proper direction. The simplest way to do this is through isolation, through muscle-setting exercise such as quad sets, straight leg raises, adductor leg raises, and standing terminal knee extensions, or TKEs. Strengthening the abductor and hip extensor muscles decreases the incidence of patellofemoral pain syndrome.

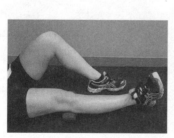
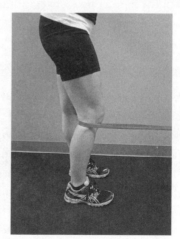

Figure 4.12

IT BAND SYNDROME

Continuing up the baseball athlete's leg, we come to the iliotibial band. Most people who have pain consistent with an IT band dysfunction complain of lateral (outside) knee pain. The IT band originates at the tensor fascia lata

(TFL) muscle (not to be confused with your favorite Starbucks beverage!) at the outside of the hip (ilium), runs along the most lateral quadriceps muscle (vastus lateralis), and inserts just below the knee joint line on the tibia.

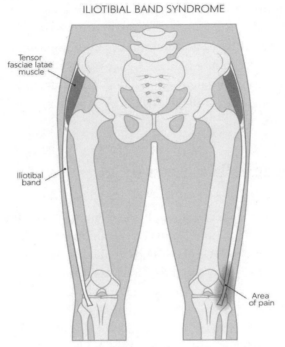

ILIOTIBIAL BAND SYNDROME

Figure 4.13

IT band syndrome (ITBS) is most commonly caused by friction between the distal IT band and the lateral femoral epicondyle, which is the bump on the outside of the knee. It is a very common injury associated with running athletes and is one of the leading causes of lateral knee pain. The tightness distending from the lateral quadricep muscle, the vastus lateralis, closes the available space between the bone and tendon, leading to increased friction while flexing and extending the knee.

Since this tendon crosses two joints, the level of debilitation can cause changes in the function of both the hip and knee when walking or running. Deviations from a normal gait pattern can lead to compensatory pain in other joints above or below the affected area.

ITBS symptoms range from a stiff joint to swelling or thickening along the entire IT band (not just around the knee). Some people describe the sensation as stinging, burning, or numbness around the knee joint, most often on the lateral side. Depending on the severity of dysfunction, this sensation can extend from the knee all the way up to the hip.

As with any inflammation, pain usually begins as mild discomfort after activity and becomes more intense over time. The pain is usually felt when the foot hits the ground and will persist in aggravation after activity. The progression of pain is typically noticed before or after activity, when moving from sitting to standing or walking up and down stairs. Once pain is present during normal daily activities, it is time to begin treatment to alleviate symptoms.

Preventing IT Band Syndrome

IT band syndrome is an overuse injury, but there are some factors that contribute to its acceleration. If an athlete trains on different levels of surface, be it downhill, uphill, or on an embankment, the body must adjust. Take a look at your street. Does it slope uphill or downhill? Or is the center of the road higher than the shoulder of the road? Consistently running the same trail or pattern will likely lead to imbalances from compensatory movements.

Muscular imbalances could be another cause of ITBS. Analysis of the lateral versus medial quadriceps muscles will likely point to an overactive lateralis, causing tightness around the IT band. Weak hip adductors could also contribute to IT band pain. A physical therapist can teach the patient how to strengthen the entire quad muscle group and help the muscles fire at a more optimal rate.

Poor training habits can also contribute to the injury. Athletes need to warm up and cool down properly, and they should not do too much, too fast, too soon.

Maintaining the flexibility of the IT band with stretching and the aid of a foam roller can prevent the onset of IT band syndrome.

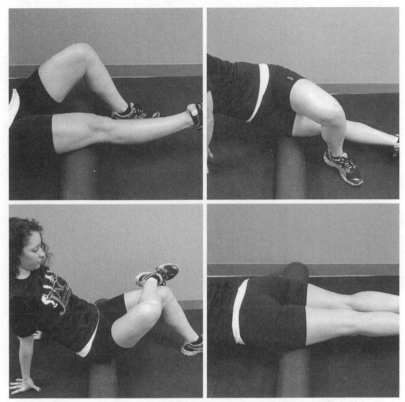

Figure 4.14

Treatment of IT Band Syndrome

It is important to remember that IT band syndrome isn't just an overuse knee injury, due to its origin at the hip. Treatment should target the joints both above and below the TFL—that is, the knee and hip—and should address the vastus lateralis muscle.

Since the primary mechanism leading to ITBS is continually flexing and extending the knee, it is important to limit or remove this causal factor. Simply take a few days off!

As with almost any injury, the first step in treating ITBS is RICE to reduce pain and inflammation (see Figure 4.3). In addition, any tight tendon should be put through a daily stretching routine to increase its internal flexibility. If proper attention is paid to ITBS at its onset, it can be managed easily. But, again, if the injury has progressed to the point where the athlete is experiencing pain with every step, along with gait changes, it is advisable to seek the attention of a medical professional.

Accomplished practitioners will use appropriate therapeutic modalities to increase circulation and decrease the inflammatory process of the fascial tissue of the tendon. As tissue pliability is restored, flexibility will increase and the downward pressure of the tendon on the knee will dissipate.

As the athlete's symptoms decrease, it is now appropriate for the physical therapist or athletic trainer to use massage, increase strengthening techniques, and progress the athlete to more functional, sport-specific exercises.

TIBIAL STRESS REACTIONS (STRESS FRACTURES AND SHIN SPLINTS)

Another common overuse injury for athletes is the stress fracture, which is a hairline crack in the bone caused by the repetitive application of force. In this case, we are talking about the tibia (shinbone), which, despite being a relatively small bone, carries 90 percent of the body's weight.

In the 19th century, stress fractures were known as "military" or "march" fractures, diagnosed in Prussian soldiers after repetitive marching. Baseball players may not be soldiers or marathoners, but base runners very often sprint on hard sand surfaces.

While most stress fractures occur when fatigued muscles can't absorb the shock of repeated impact and subsequently transfer the stress of the load to the bone, some also arise through an innate weakness in the bone, often due to conditions such as osteoporosis.

Stress fractures typically result as a progression of medial tibial stress syndrome, or shin splints. Shin splints occur when the muscle pulls away from its attachment to the tibia. When the muscle is not there as an absorption tool, the bone primarily absorbs the force.

Bone stress fractures occur when there is an imbalance between how much we are breaking down and how much we are rebuilding on a daily basis. If we break down more than we rebuild, the structure will ultimately fail.

Signs and Symptoms of Tibial Stress Reactions

A tibial stress reaction is felt in the lower part of the shin, primarily on the medial (inner) side. Early onset pain is generally noticed during activity, and progresses to bouts of pain after activity. Often, a hot spot or tender spot will develop along the shin, and will be felt by the athlete when palpating along the length of the bone.

The only true way for a medical professional to diagnose shin splints or a stress fracture is with an X-ray, bone scan, or MRI. If the fracture is large enough to be seen on an X-ray, the athlete will have been in considerable pain for a long time. Often, X-rays can identify evidence of bone healing, indicative of a stress reaction.

Causes of Tibial Stress Reaction

Some of the causes of a stress fracture can be poor biomechanics, flat feet or fallen arches, inflexible or weak muscles, improper shoes, training and playing excessively on hard surfaces, eating disorders, low calcium levels or, as I keep saying, too much too soon!

Preventing stress fractures, then, also relies on a well-balanced diet, including vitamin D, and making sure we are training with the appropriate equipment.

How to Treat Tibial Stress Reactions

There are many schools of thought about treating stress fractures in the sports medicine world. I believe if you continue to run on a small fracture, it will eventually develop into a full fracture, which will effectively put you on the sideline for eight to ten weeks.

Again, we go back to early recognition. Due to the difficulty of differentiating between a stress fracture and a shin splint, it is a good idea to stop activity and see a health-care professional as soon as shin pain is felt.

With shin splints and stress fractures in the lower leg, it is also important to remember that rest may not only mean taking a break from running and playing baseball. The standing and walking we do to complete normal, daily activities can often be too much for a bone that has been stressed.

It may be necessary to put the athlete in a walking boot, air cast, or full lower leg air cast for four to eight weeks, and up to sixteen to twenty weeks if the injury progresses to a full fracture.

Whether the injury requires immobilization or not, it is important that the athlete be pain-free prior to beginning any strengthening or aerobic activity.

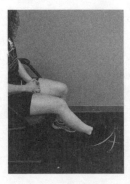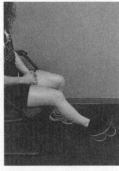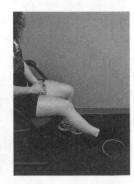

Figure 4.15

Once pain-free, **Phase One** of recovery is restoring range of motion. The ankle joint must have full range of motion before functional training can begin. In addition, lower leg muscle flexibility will help long-term by allowing for more shock absorption in the lower extremity during running and training.

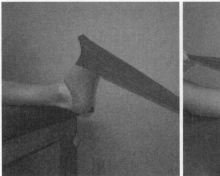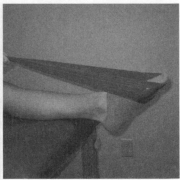

Figure 4.16

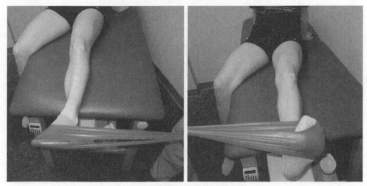

Figure 4.16

Phase Two is to begin low-level, low-impact strengthening. This might include four-way ankle exercises for the shin, ankle, and foot muscles, including the gastroc-soleus complex and anterior tibialis.

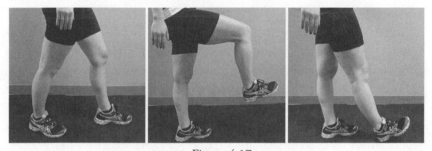

Figure 4.17

Finally, **Phase Three** of rehab will progress the athlete into functional and full weight-bearing activities. As with any injury, there is no direct route from the training table back to the diamond. Athletes must recover their general fitness and then gradually progress to a full return to play.

BURSITIS

The last of the overuse injuries we will discuss is bursitis. Between our muscles, tendons, and bones are small bursal sacs of synovial fluid, the body's lubricant. These sacs act as cushions and help joints move more fluidly by reducing friction between tendons and bones.

Synovial joint of the knee

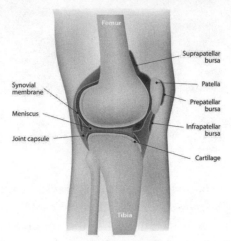

Figure 4.18

Bursa sacs in any joint can become inflamed, but this generally occurs in response to specific motions that are repeated over time. A simple way to imagine this is to picture stretching a rubber band and rubbing it against the side of a desk. The rubber band will eventually tear from the friction that is generated. Now imagine placing a small bladder of liquid in between the rubber band and the desk. This would decrease the amount of friction generated between the desk and the band (or bone and tendon) by acting as a buffer between the two surfaces. But with repeated trauma, even the bursa sac can become inflamed.

Another factor is the internal extensibility, or flexibility, of the tendon, or the tendon's ability to be stretched. As we continue with our rubber band example, think about the different types of bands. Some are short and thick and have little extensibility, while others are long and thin and have greater extensibility.

When these bursa sacs become inflamed, it causes pain and stiffness with simple flexion and extension. Depending on the severity, there may be a huge amount of inflammation around the joint. The most common types of lower extremity bursitis in baseball players are:

- Pre-patellar, at the front of the knee
- Infra-patellar, below your kneecap

- Trochanteric, at the hip bone
- Achilles, at the calf tendon
- Iliopsoas, at the front of the hip
- Ischial, at the buttocks (those two bones you sit on all day long)

Underlying factors, such as rheumatoid arthritis, can contribute to bursitis, but it is most commonly a result of overuse. It can also result from trauma from a fall, most commonly in the buttocks, hip, or knee. As with any fluid-filled sac, a direct blow to the bursa has the ability to rupture it. When this happens, there is generally a large amount of extra-articular swelling, or swelling outside of the joint. Oftentimes, the joint itself is not maximally inhibited, and much of the joint's function remains intact.

If infection is suspected, the athlete must be examined by a physician immediately for an appropriate diagnosis. Some common signs and symptoms of an infected bursa sac include:

- Erythema (redness)
- Swelling
- Emitting heat, or is warm to the touch
- Increased pain and tenderness

Advanced bursitis results in a very red, swollen, stiff, painful joint. Some patients have even described it as "a big ball of redness."

How to Prevent Bursitis

By looking at the way forces are distributed across the tendon, bursa, and bone, we can define ways to limit the amount of force and friction generated between these tissues. By increasing the flexibility of the surrounding musculature, we can decrease the amount of pressure generated over time with repetitive actions.

How to Treat Bursitis

Throughout the therapeutic process, the goal is to decrease the inflammation of the bursa, while increasing the flexibility of the tendon.

As the inflammation of the bursa decreases, the stiffness in the joint will also decrease.

Bursitis will usually resolve itself in seven to ten days with good therapeutic management, and the athlete can return to sport quite rapidly as long as swelling around the joint has been eliminated.

If a physician suspects a potential infection, he or she may prescribe an antibiotic. If the bursitis becomes chronic, the physician may perform an aspiration, or physical removal of the fluid with a syringe. In severe cases, the inflamed or infected bursa may also be removed surgically. If this course of action is needed, it will likely lead to more problems down the road, especially for the running athlete, and possibly involving a surgical tendon repair.

Once again, a minor problem of inflexibility can develop into a deeper issue involving multiple tissues, if left untreated. To achieve every baseball player's goal of staying on the diamond or mound, early intervention is key!

CHAPTER 5
by Dr. Christopher Ahmad

SHOULDER INJURIES

The shoulder is at risk for injury and tissue breakdown because of the delicate balance required to stably center the ball within the socket while maintaining a tremendous range of motion. As mentioned in Chapter 1, repetitive and enormous arm rotation speed coupled with tremendous joint force pushes the shoulder toward injury.

MECHANISM OF INJURY THEORIES

Three main theories that now guide treatment have gained acceptance to explain why baseball players injure their shoulders: the internal impingement theory, the posterior capsular contracture theory, and the scapulothoracic function theory. The internal impingement theory explains direct injury to anatomic structures such as SLAP tears (superior labral tear from anterior to posterior), biceps injuries, and rotator cuff injuries. The posterior capsular contracture theory explains how loss of internal shoulder rotation with muscle strength imbalances can cause injury. Lastly, the scapulothoracic function theory explains how biomechanical factors, including kinetic chain deficits and scapular motion alterations, can lead to injury. While it is helpful to divide the causes of a disabled shoulder into various groups, shoulder pathology in the throwing athlete should be viewed as a continuum of interrelated problems and may include aspects of all the theories.

Internal Impingement Theory

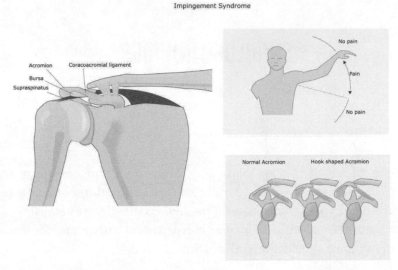

Figure 5.1

Internal impingement describes the shoulder position in the cocking phase of throwing. This is when the external rotation of the shoulder is maxed out and the rotator cuff makes contact with the glenoid labrum. This contact is regarded as a normal arm movement process. However, forceful and repeated contact causes partial thickness rotator cuff tears and superior labral tears. For many athletes, this repeated contact and the associated tears do not cause pain. In fact, the tear patterns may give the thrower better motion and even improve throwing. However, at some point, the degree of change to the rotator cuff and/or the labrum can cause symptoms. Several factors can increase the force of the internal impingement contact, increasing tear size risk. One factor is improper mechanics, with the elbow moving posterior to the body, which often occurs in an attempt to compensate for lower extremity issues in the kinetic chain. The natural impingement can be escalated to become pathologic with excessive force at the contact site. This results in rotator cuff and labral tearing. Another factor occurs when the anterior capsule is stretched, allowing the humeral head to move forward relative to the socket, thereby increasing the contact force.

Rotator Cuff Muscles

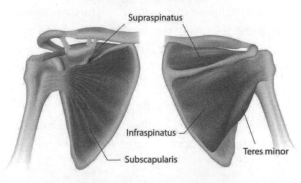

Figure 5.2

<u>Posterior Capsular Contracture Theory</u>

The posterior capsule is comprised of the ligaments in the back of the shoulder, adding stability to the ball and socket joint. This capsule must withstand forces up to 150 pounds during the deceleration and follow-through phases of throwing. Repetitive forces can cause inflammation, scarring, and contraction of those soft tissues, at which time the shoulder does not rotate normally. The contracted soft tissue acts to tether shoulder motion and shifts the ball away from the socket during rotation. Shifting the ball within the socket can create increased force on the labrum and rotator cuff, causing injury. "Glenohumeral internal rotation deficit" is a term thrown around by physical therapists, athletic trainers, and physicians involved with baseball health. This refers to loss of motion in the shoulder where greater than 20 degrees of internal rotation is lost compared to the contralateral side and the throwing shoulder. This may or may not be associated with greater external rotation. It is important to have adequate total range of motion because as much as a 5-degree loss of range of motion increases the likelihood of injuring your throwing shoulder up to two to three times.

Scapulothoracic Function Theory

The scapula or wing blade plays a vital role in transferring energy from the trunk to the humerus during overhead throwing, and every coach and player should know its importance. The scapula must move in concert with the shoulder during throwing. Weakness of the scapular muscles can disrupt this relationship and alter the forces transmitted to the shoulder girdle. If the scapula is out of position, the socket can exacerbate internal impingement forces. Having studied the changes in scapula positioning in throwers, I have found the scapula rotated inward with lessened mobility along the thoracic wall.

Injury to the throwing shoulder can present as a cascade of pathologic events and can be quite complex. Poor throwing mechanics, such as weak force generation in the trunk, or abnormal shoulder positioning such as hyper-external rotation, can cause microtrauma to the rotator cuff and labrum. This complex process leading to shoulder injury is often considered a continuum because the interplay among the various components can compound and escalate the risk leading to injury.

THE THROWING SHOULDER

Asymptomatic Throwing Shoulder Adaptation

An emerging and important concept is that baseball players develop necessary adaptive changes to their throwing shoulders. During development, especially during adolescence, the throwing shoulder undergoes several adaptations compared to its opposite shoulder, including increased external rotation. My research demonstrates that throwers can externally rotate their shoulders to a much higher degree than their non-throwing shoulder. We also discovered that these changes take place during adolescence, occurring in bone and soft tissues around the shoulder.

The bone of the upper arm is called the proximal humerus. Many throwing athletes show widening of the growth plate while young. This stress to the growth plate, usually around age thirteen to fourteen, changes the shape of the bone to where the ball is rotated more toward the back of the body. The result is that the arm also rotates more toward the back, or it can externally rotate. In addition, the socket may developmentally face slightly more toward the back of the shoulder, allowing increased external rotation. It is theorized that this rotation is an adaptation that allows external rotation and, at the same time, limits the internal rotation of the shoulder. In addition, the capsule tissue that helps provide stability for the shoulder becomes more lax in the front of the shoulder and stiffer in the back, which also increases external rotation.

What's interesting is that, at birth, we are able to rotate the shoulder externally. The humerus bone is positioned with the ball facing more toward the back of the body and, with growth, the ball changes its position. This is somewhat interrupted during adolescence with repetitive throwing. Increased external shoulder rotation is now thought to be a healthy feature for mature athletes, as there will be less forceful internal impingement with hard throwing and fewer injuries.

MRI Scans and the Throwing Shoulder

It is often said that, if a baseball player wants to avoid surgery, never ever get an MRI scan of the shoulder. The reason is that asymptomatic professional baseball players who are pitching effectively and without pain have numerous abnormalities on MRI scans. In fact, up to 80 percent of baseball players can have an abnormal labrum. In addition, MRI scans will show as many as 50 percent of players without symptoms having partial or full thickness rotator cuff tears. Why is there so much abnormality when patients aren't having symptoms? The reason is as we have discussed regarding the theories of pathomechanics of the shoulder. There is a natural contact of the rotator cuff against the labrum and, to achieve the external rotation and required motion of the shoulder, there can be partial tears of the rotator cuff, as well as perceived injury to the labrum, where these injury features are really simply adaptive changes.

Young players often appear in my office with MRI scans in their hands that show abnormalities causing extreme concern. First, the MRI reports that describe extreme pathology suggest that the child will never throw a baseball again. Secondly, parents believe that, if tissue is damaged or torn, it must be fixed to get back to hard throwing. Physicians, therefore, need to properly educate and reassure their patients and families. Abnormalities on MRI scans are so common that we often call them "normal findings of the throwing shoulder." I use the analogy that hitters develop calluses on their hands, which is normal for a hitter, and throwers develop changes in the rotator cuff and the labrum, which is normal for a thrower. I occasionally have patients being evaluated for tumors in their shoulder based on MRI and, more often it is simply abnormal signal in the humerus bone from the internal impingement process. This can certainly be scary for patients and families.

If there are symptoms, however, the exact cause must be determined. The baseball athlete, unlike those who play other sports, requires the expertise of a skilled sports medicine specialist to determine the exact source of pain in the shoulder. This comes from a thorough and experienced evaluation of symptoms, the patient's history, and a physical examination, in addition to the MRI. It's important for patients to know that an MRI can show tears and pathologies and inflammation. But the MRI does not allow a physician to see or conclude where pain is coming from. More simply, you cannot see pain on the MRI.

ROTATOR CUFF TEARS

The rotator cuff is essential to stable motion of the shoulder. It is comprised of four muscles that attach from the scapula to the humerus. The rotator cuff can tear, inflame, or both.

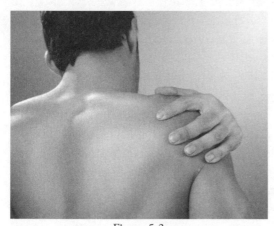

Figure 5.3

Signs and Symptoms of Rotator Cuff Tears

Important symptoms that guide treatment include the location and severity of pain. Rotator cuff tears and inflammation cause pain in the back-top and back-front of the shoulder. Often, players will feel their arm is dead when trying to throw. They experience pain when their arm is in the late cocking phase of throwing (see Figure 1.4) and, with worsening symptoms, patients can have pain with routine activities and even lose sleep because of shoulder soreness. Examination by a physician, athletic trainer, or other medical specialist will uncover weakness of the rotator cuff, as well as signs of impingement. The examiner performs these indirectly, putting pressure and contact on the rotator cuff. When injured, the sensitive, inflamed, or torn rotator cuff causes pain with these maneuvers.

Finally, an MRI can be used to determine the status of the rotator cuff. However, as emphasized previously, the rotator cuff is often abnormal on the MRI, and it should not be used in isolation to guide treatment. It is critically important that medical professionals taking care of baseball players know how to perform a skillful history and physical exam to make the correct diagnosis.

Treating Rotator Cuff Tears

Treatment for rotator cuff tears on a throwing athlete always begins non-operatively. The goal is to first reduce inflammation through a period of rest, use of anti-inflammatory medication, and modalities. This phase of treatment is followed by motion restoration of the rotator cuff, then periscapular muscle strengthening. As a player becomes symptom-free and shoulder strength is restored, lower extremity and core strengthening is emphasized. Then, a throwing program can be initiated. It's important for parents and coaches to know that it takes time for non-operative treatment to work. Often, this can take up to three to six months.

For patients unable to get back to their desired level of throwing, surgery may be indicated to allow them their best chance. Most shoulder pathology in the throwing athlete can be treated arthroscopically. Surgical treatment for rotator cuff tears in throwing athletes can take one of three options. It should be noted that the results of surgery for a damaged rotator cuff are generally poor when compared to other surgical procedures on baseball players. For example, professional and competitive athletes in some studies were able to return to play only 35 percent of the time. While other studies show more encouraging results, with return to play upwards of 85 percent, it is still a major concern, and most physicians who are knowledgeable in the care of baseball athletes choose surgery as the final phase of an algorithm.

Often, season and career timing influence the decision for surgery even more than the tear itself. For example, a collegiate scholarship athlete with disabling symptoms at the end of the season may choose earlier surgical intervention as opposed to another athlete who is not as pressured to get back to playing quickly.

Why are the results of rotator cuff surgery so poor? The answer is unclear. We do appreciate that the rotator cuff is an extremely essential dynamic stabilizer of the shoulder and, when compromised, can cause symptoms. At the same time, the rotator cuff undergoes adaptive changes, including partial thickness tears. Therefore, the fine line between normal rotator cuff changes and pathologic rotator cuff injury is unclear for throwing athletes. This also raises questions on the best surgical treatment. Reconnecting the tendon to bone may tether the compensatory anatomy of the rotator cuff and lead to less than ideal outcomes. Often, the best outcome is when the surgeon takes a minimalist approach to dealing with partial rotator cuff tears. This may be to create a surgical repair that prevents progression of a tear without limiting the significant range of motion required for competitive play.

SLAP LESIONS AND LABRAL TEARS

I performed a study that showed a shocking trend of SLAP (superior labral tear from anterior to posterior) repair surgery increasing in New York state: from 2002 to 2009, we observed a 250 percent increase of SLAP tear procedures. The reason for the increase is not clear, but it is definitely happening. A controversy currently exists regarding the treatment of SLAP lesions and baseball players. SLAP lesions are extremely common and must be confirmed as the source of symptoms before beginning treatment.

Signs and Symptoms of SLAP Lesions and Labral Tears

A wide spectrum of disorders other than specific shoulder complaints may be present in the thrower and should be investigated. These include downstream disorders of the kinetic chain, such as issues with the core, lower back, and hips. Initial shoulder symptoms are often not pain-related, but, rather, complaints of decreased control, velocity, and difficulty warming up.

Patients will often not be able to recall a specific inciting event, but, rather, note that their symptoms developed gradually over time. They may also present with symptoms similar to rotator cuff disease, such as a "dead arm," or shoulder weakness after throwing. Patients may also describe popping, snapping, and locking, which may occur with unstable labral tears. As a result of excessive anterior capsular laxity and rotator cuff dysfunction, patients may say that their shoulder feels unstable and is "slipping out" while throwing. Athletes with posterosuperior impingement often complain of shoulder pain during the late cocking phase of throwing. While the pain is typically localized to the posterior aspect of the shoulder, it may also be more generalized.

A thorough and systematic physical examination of the thrower must include an assessment of the lower back, hips, and knees. Single leg squats are useful for the evaluation of hip and trunk control, muscle balance, and flexibility. The physical examination of the shoulder always begins visually, noting the patient's posture and general appearance, and how the patient ambulates and moves the shoulder. Inspection begins with assessing the skin for any scars, either from prior surgery or from prior trauma. Subsequently, with the patient facing away from the clinician, the clinician must look for any evidence of asymmetry between the shoulders, as well as for potential signs of atrophy and scapular winging.

Range of motion of both shoulders should be tested in both adduction and 90 degrees of abduction. The thrower will usually have decreased internal rotation and increased external rotation, while maintaining the total arc of motion. Strength testing should isolate the muscle being tested. Since there is a strong association between internal impingement and SLAP lesions, clinical testing should coincide with these suspicions. The active compression test has high sensitivity and specificity for SLAP lesions that are causing symptoms. The examiner positions the arm and asks the patient to resist downward pressure. This will cause pressure to be applied internally to the labrum. A torn labrum will elicit pain with this maneuver.

Treating SLAP Lesions and Labral Tears

Non-operative treatment should follow a sequential, progressive, three-phased approach that highlights the entire kinetic chain while restoring glenohumeral joint mobility/soft tissue extensibility. This is detailed more in Chapter 3. The first, acute, phase should restore this muscular activation by promoting synchronous muscle firing when demands on the tissue are relatively low. Anti-inflammatory strategies are employed to combat soft tissue irritation while restoring glenohumeral motion necessary for overhead throwing. The second, recovery, phase, emphasizes kinetic chain linkage through resistance training to the core, lower extremity, and trunk. Phase Three, the functional phase, imparts sport-specific, functional movement patterns necessary for a return to throwing. Plyometric exercise, shoulder end-range stabilization drills, and advanced isotonic strengthening are key components before initiating a throwing program and eventual return to sport. Exercises during this phase are endurance-based with a propensity toward high repetition and low resistance.

Surgical treatment is indicated for patients who have failed nonsurgical management and who accept the associated risks. Although the results of operative treatment do improve symptoms after surgery, the prognosis of returning to asymptomatic throwing and the prior level of performance is guarded. For this reason, we recommend that the throwing athlete undergo an initial period of a guided therapy regimen before surgical intervention. Due to the "normal" adaptive changes of the throwing shoulder, surgical intervention should be entertained with a "less is more" approach. Any surgical intervention should be aimed at recreating the anatomy inherent to the throwing shoulder, and, in cases of intraoperative decision-making, a minimalist approach often provides superior outcomes over aggressive surgical intervention.

SLAP repair is performed arthroscopically. Our current preferred technique is to securely reattach the labrum back to the socket using strong fixation that is low profile. The outcome of SLAP repair in elite overhead-throwing (e.g., racquet sports, volleyball) athletes is sobering. Certain studies show returned play at approximately 60 percent in cases of just SLAP repair without rotator cuff disease. However, it can be as high as 80 percent in players with both SLAP lesion and a partial thickness rotator cuff repair. This indicates that rotator cuff pathology is a major contributing factor to failure of SLAP treatment.

There is interest in a procedure called biceps tenodesis for throwing athletes because, in the case of a failed SLAP repair, a biceps tenodesis can be beneficial. The procedure involves cutting the bicep, which attaches to the superior labrum, and reattaching it at a different location. This takes the stress off the labrum, which can contribute to the etiology and pathology of the pain. Because many athletes benefit from bicep tenodesis and the recovery time is less than for the SLAP repair, bicep tenodesis is an evolving treatment option for many athletes desiring more rapid recovery or treatment for a SLAP repair that did not relieve symptoms.

CHAPTER 6
by Dr. Christopher Ahmad

TOMMY JOHN SURGERY AND OTHER ELBOW INJURIES

Tommy John's record of 13-3 included five complete games and three shutouts back in mid-season, 1974. John, pitching for the Los Angeles Dodgers, was working out of trouble and attempted a sinker to produce a double play during a game against the Montreal Expos, and the pain was immediate and searing in his elbow. Without MRI technology available, Doctor Frank Jobe diagnosed John with an elbow ulnar collateral ligament tear solely based on a physical examination and X-rays. Jobe put John's arm in a cast for four weeks, hoping that the UCL would heal, but it became clear that the injury would not heal on its own. Unable to pitch, and unwilling to give up, John instructed Jobe to surgically fix his elbow. The challenge was that a surgical solution was nonexistent. Jobe was aware of tendon grafts being used in hand surgery and designed and executed an ulnar collateral ligament reconstruction with palmaris longus autograft to recreate the UCL. He passed the graft through tunnels he drilled in the bones of the elbow and sewed the graft in place. After two years of rehabilitation, John resumed pitching.

Fourteen seasons and 164 wins later, John retired at age 46. Following John's successful outcome, Jobe went on to directly help the careers of hundreds of pitchers with his surgery and, indirectly, the surgeons he taught the procedure to, who then went on to perform the surgery.

SIGNS AND SYMPTOMS – WHAT TO LOOK OUT FOR

I reviewed game film on Chase Whitley playing against the Tampa Bay Rays. And, to the naked eye of an orthopedic surgeon, nothing in his pitching motion could be identified to cause injury to his elbow And, yet, he waved to the training staff and eventually walked off the mound and made his way to the training room. The evening of the injury, I received a call that Chase had a suspected UCL tear. This is comparable to ligament injury in other sports, such as when a soccer player stops and cuts, and then video shows the knee buckling out of position and the player collapsing to the ground—or a football player who dislocates his shoulder when tackled. In fact, in my research, I have reviewed film on numerous MLB players to learn the pitching mechanics associated with Tommy John injury. There is nothing obvious to the naked eye, because the tearing of the ligament is not a singular event. The tearing was a process of repeated stresses to the ligament, like a wire hanger being bent back and forth. Finally, it breaks, with little effort creating the final bend.

Patients who injure their UCL have various symptoms. The injury most commonly afflicts high-level athletes involved in intense throwing. It's important to ascertain the position, competitive level, and future aspirations of athletes who have injured their ligament to determine proper treatment. It's also important to ascertain a sudden difference in the volume of throwing, pitching mechanics, or the velocity of throwing. Patients may also have a history of a problem with their hip, leg, or core, such as injury or inflexibility that could have contributed to their injury.

Symptoms specific to the elbow should be ascertained, such as degree and exact location of pain. It occurs during throwing, especially in the acceleration phase, and any associated symptoms, such as numbness and tingling in the fingers or pain in the back of the elbow or locking or catching, should be noted. UCL injury encompasses a spectrum of symptoms. On one end, the player may feel a sudden pop of acute pain on the inside of the elbow during a game and be unable to continue throwing. On the other end of the spectrum, a patient may simply have progressive loss of accuracy and the ability to loosen up and throw with diminishing velocity.

The inside aspect of the elbow demonstrates swelling or tenderness to palpation overlying the ligament range. Range of motion may be limited.

Ulnar Collateral Ligament

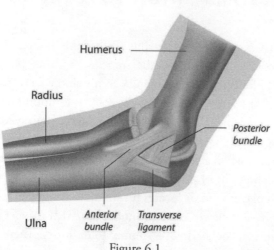

Humerus

Radius

Posterior bundle

Ulna

Anterior bundle

Transverse ligament

Figure 6.1

The hallmark test to indicate a ligament tear is called "the moving valgus stress test." The examiner stabilizes the elbow against an exam table and puts subtle stress across the arm, which pulls on the UCL. Patients with a UCL tear experience pain as the elbow is flexed and extended. Patients with a suspected UCL injury typically undergo X-rays as the initial imaging study. X-rays may demonstrate loose bodies of bone spurs and even arthritis in the elbow. To fully diagnose a UCL injury accurately, an MRI enables detection of partial thickness tears or full thickness tears. Occasionally, dye contrast is injected into the elbow when a standard MRI is inconclusive.

HOW TO TREAT UCL TEARS

Treatment requires careful consideration of the patient's athletic expectations in addition to the degree of UCL injury. Also important is seasonal and career timing. On the one hand, athletes with low demands who are less serious about continuing with baseball may choose to play first base rather than a high-demand position, such as pitching, as they undergo non-operative treatment, which is initially favored in this setting. Players who are serious, perhaps with aspirations of playing at the professional level, may opt for more immediate surgical reconstruction.

Initial non-operative treatment for UCL injury consists of rest, ice, anti-inflammatory medication, and, in some cases, use of a brace. This is aimed at reducing pain and inflammation and allowing initial healing. We highly discourage cortisone injections into the area of the UCL. The use of platelet-rich plasma (PRP) has gained popularity recently. In fact, I perform close to one hundred PRP injections into the UCL of athletes of all levels of play each year.

PLATELET-RICH PLASMA THERAPY

Platelet-rich plasma therapy, a treatment to aid the regeneration of ligament and tendon injuries, is shortening rehabilitation time and often eliminates the need for surgery. Platelet-rich plasma therapy is part of a relatively new field of medicine known as orthobiologics that includes the use of stem cells and emphasizes the latest technologies along with the body's natural ability to heal itself. Blood is made of red blood cells, white blood cells, plasma, and platelets. Platelet-rich plasma (PRP) is the name given to blood plasma with a high concentration of platelets that contains huge doses of bioactive proteins, such as growth factors, that are critical in the repair and regeneration of tissues. To extract these platelets, a small amount of blood is drawn from the patient and immediately undergoes centrifugation, a process by which mixtures are separated using centripetal force. This process separates out red blood cells, which carry oxygen, and the platelet and the plasma. The platelets with the plasma have all the healing agents. Once we've done the separation, we extract the platelet-rich plasma, and it can then be injected back into the patient's injured area. It is their own platelet-rich plasma—it isn't taken from another person or developed in a laboratory.

Growth factors can dramatically enhance tissue recovery, and the special proteins also initiate new blood vessel formation, bone regeneration and healing, connective tissue repair, and wound healing. There is little chance for rejection because the components used for treatment are extracted from a person's own body. This makes the procedure entirely safe. The PRP injection also carries less chance for infection than an incision, with a considerably shorter recovery time than after surgery.

I began using PRP therapy as an option for professional athletes. Once we established that this approach was beneficial for the professional, I began offering it to young athletes. We have an even greater motivation to use a healing agent for younger patients. The younger a patient is, the less we want to operate, which is potentially career-ending if it doesn't work, or could possibly change the normal anatomy. We try to preserve a patient's own anatomy and tissues and avoid surgery as much as possible.

I have researched the effects of injury in younger children and adolescents as compared to adults. Preliminary data shows that a sports injury in an adolescent has much greater impact on his or her emotional status and perception of quality of life. That makes sense because adults work and have other responsibilities. With students, their focus and energy are on school, socializing and, often, athletics. If you take away their ability to be involved in athletics, it affects their school and social environment. Young athletes have so much future potential, and if we don't provide the maximum benefit to them, they have a long life to feel the repercussions.

As Director of Biomechanics Research at the Center for Orthopaedic Research, I continue to explore the uses and benefits of PRP. We know that the platelet-rich plasma is working, but what we aren't sure about yet is what the exact dosing should be. Is one injection enough? Are two injections better? Are three injections too many? So I'm involved in determining what the exact dose should be. Major League Baseball funded an ongoing study to determine the effects of repeated dosing and optimal timing between doses.

I conducted a study with several colleagues to evaluate the effect of PRP injections on partial UCL tears in high-level throwing athletes. We reviewed the results of forty-four baseball players (six professional, fourteen college, and twenty-four high school) treated with PRP injections for partial-thickness UCL tears. Mean age was 17.3 years. Of the forty-four patients, fifteen (34 percent) had an excellent outcome, seventeen had a good outcome, two had a fair outcome, and ten had a poor outcome. After injection, four (67 percent) of the six professional players returned to professional play. There were no injection-related complications. Our use of PRP in the treatment of UCL insufficiency produced outcomes much better than previous outcomes from conservative treatment of these injuries. PRP injections may be particularly beneficial in young athletes who have sustained acute damage to an isolated part of the ligament and in athletes unwilling or unable to undergo the extended rehabilitation required after surgical reconstruction of the ligament.

The period of rest with non-operative treatment with or without PRP is typically six weeks. That includes a period of global strengthening with particular emphasis on the rotator cuff in the periscapular muscles. When the elbow examination is back to normal with no tenderness in the negative stress test, then a throwing program can be initiated. Throwing mechanics are optimized, and flexibility and strength is maintained in the lower extremities, trunk, and core. The total time for non-operative treatment before a player is back to playing competitively is typically three to four months. Patients should continue to avoid overuse when back to playing with no simultaneous participation in sports with similar motions, e.g., tennis or swimming.

Patients who wish to continue baseball, but fail non-operative treatments, and maintain symptoms and the ability to throw, are indicated for Tommy John surgery. Tommy John surgery requires a long and lengthy recovery, which is demanding both physically and mentally, and the patient and the other athletes need a full commitment to the process to achieve a great result.

SURGICAL TECHNIQUES

UCL Repair

The UCL can often be repaired if the injured ligament is of overall good quality and it is injured in a discrete area. But, patient selection is important. The best patients are young athletes with avulsion-type injuries where the remainder of the ligament is healthy outside the zone of injury. In addition, the recovery time for UCL repair with an internal brace system is accelerated compared to a standard Tommy John surgery. Patients with extreme seasonal timing issues, such as a high school or college player wishing to play a final season, with at least six months before the season starts, may elect such treatment.

The surgical technique involves making an incision over the inside aspect of the elbow. The dissection is then performed to expose the ligament tear, which is fully evaluated to confirm that a repair technique is suitable for the tear pattern in that situation. Next, a suture anchor, which is a device to anchor suture material to bone, is put in place. The sutures are passed through the tear of the ligament and tied, fixating the injury. Next, an internal brace, which is attached to the suture anchor, similar to a shoelace, is created to take the stress off the repair. The ends of the shoelace-type material are then fixed across the elbow joint, thereby absorbing the stress like suspenders. Following surgery, the rehab includes a brief period of immobilization, followed by a range of motion exercises for strengthening. A throwing program can begin ten weeks after surgery, and progressive throwing is performed until the patient is game-ready, which may be six months, following surgery.

Tommy John Surgery Technique

Tommy John surgery begins with an incision over the inside aspect of the elbow. The dissection is carried through tissues until the UCL is fully exposed. The UCL tear is confirmed, and then reconstruction is carried out. First, drill tunnels are created at the precise locations on the bone where the UCL naturally attaches. Once the bone tunnels are created and connected, the graft is obtained either from the wrist with the tendon called the "palmaris longus" or the knee. Twenty percent of people do not have a palmaris longus at their wrist, and removal of this tendon does not influence the ability to return to throwing. Patients who have either a very small palmaris longus or don't have one at all typically have the graft taken from their knee. Once the graft is obtained and cleaned, the free end has high-strength sutures placed in it. The graft is then woven through the bone tunnels and secured in place with sutures. Variations in surgical technique usually involve how the graft is fixed within the tunnels. One method to fix the graft is to suture the graft side to side. Another method is to use a docking technique where the graft is controlled with sutures, docked into a tunnel, and tied over a bone bridge. Another method is to have the sutures controlling the graft sutured into the native ligament.

Approximately 80 percent of my practice involves the docking technique; however, I've made special modifications to this technique to get at least three or four strands of graft across the elbow. This creates a larger ligament, which, in theory, will be more durable.

Recovery from Tommy John Surgery

The rehabilitation following Tommy John surgery is challenging. The goal is for the graft to obtain a natural blood supply and convert it to the exact properties of a native ligament. This process has been termed *ligamentization*. During this biologic healing, incremental increases in stress are applied to the ligament. Approximately one year is required for the graft tissue to assume the new function. However, it's becoming clear that even additional time is beneficial, and the average time for a professional Major League pitcher to get back to his level of competition is sixteen to eighteen months. In addition to addressing ligament healing, the entire upper and lower extremity is enhanced.

The timeline for the protocol is from zero to ten days, following surgery. A splint is worn for two to six weeks, while progressive range-of-motion exercises of the elbow and shoulder are performed with light resistance exercises beginning with the forearm and shoulder. At sixteen weeks, the athlete should have full range of motion. From two to four months, aggressive resistance exercises of the entire upper extremity, including the rotator cuff and the lower body and trunk, are conditioned. At four to five months, if the patient demonstrates excellent strength, full range of motion, and no tenderness, a throwing program is initiated, throwing three times a week, progressing from sixty to ninety to 120 feet and, in some instances, beyond 120 feet. At nine to ten months, a mound program is started for pitchers with low throw effort and straight pitches off the mound. They then progress to throwing full effort and breaking pitches. The pitcher will then progress into game situations, initially throwing batting practice and then low-number pitches and games.

Return to Play

On average, I think athletes should be back to competition in twelve months. They might be sent down to a Minor League rehab assignment, or it might be offseason, but if a Major League player has surgery in July, the fans can expect him to be back next July. However, his stats won't be as good that first year. Most pitchers are able to make a full recovery from UCL reconstruction, but the road back is a long and difficult one. The timeline ranges from twelve to eighteen months and involves a series of incremental steps. Although the surgery has not changed much in the forty-plus years since Jobe first pioneered it, the understanding of how to rehab the elbow has greatly evolved.

Anticipated Outcomes

Following John's initial success, reports have been extremely encouraging. Many surgeons report their outcomes are 80 to 90 percent successful in return to play, including pitching. Negative factors for return have been identified, which most often relate to other injuries along with the UCL injury. Some examples include tearing of the forearm muscle, cartilage injury, and revision or second-time surgery.

VALGUS EXTENSION OVERLOAD AND POSTEROMEDIAL IMPINGEMENT

Almost everyone in the baseball community has heard of bone chips in the elbow that require removal. In fact, it is extremely common at the end of the baseball season for professional athletes to seek this treatment. Bone chips are created by repetitive stress across the elbow and have been recognized for close to one hundred years. Personally, I have been involved in numerous studies that generated widely accepted conclusions.

In the follow-through phase of throwing, the elbow extends rapidly and the articular cartilage and bone in the back of the elbow experience enormous force. The bone responds to the force by growing spurs or extra bone, similar to how skin forms a callus from repetitive baseball bat swinging. At some point, the bone spurs can crack and create intense pain. A small cracked spur in the elbow can create pain similar to a pebble beneath your heel in your shoe. Often, these bone spurs form more rapidly when a player has a slightly loose UCL. In fact, I studied this in the laboratory with cadavers, where we put pressure-sensitive film into the elbows and modified the laxity of the ligament. Increasing laxity of the UCL caused more stress in the exact area that bone spurs develop, proving the hypothesis that looseness in the ligament may contribute to the formation of bone chips in patients. This is extremely important because removing spurs may take place in the setting of an injured ligament. And it's common clinically to see athletes develop the need for UCL reconstruction following bone spur removal.

It's also clear that surgical removal of more than just bone spurs or extra bone in the back of the elbow will increase stress on the ligament. It was once common practice for surgeons to remove aggressive amounts of bone with the thought that this would stop bone reforming. I studied strain gauges on the UCL. With increasing amounts of bone removal, the strain on the ligament increased. It is, therefore, my clinical recommendation to surgeons performing this operation to remove only the damaged bone and preserve as much normal bone as possible.

Signs and Symptoms of Bone Chips

Likely candidates are heavy throwers playing baseball, for example, but it may also occur with other sports such as tennis, softball, football, and lacrosse. The pain is localized to the back of the elbow. It's often associated with decreased velocity and control. Often, mechanical symptoms, such as catching or elbow locking, may be experienced with loose bone chips getting stuck in the joint. Players will have difficulty warming up. It's important to note whether they have any history of prior UCL injury that may indicate a looseness or laxity in the UCL.

Examination reveals decreased extension of the elbow and tenderness in the back part of the elbow. Quickly snapping the elbow into extension causes the patient pain. X-rays often demonstrate bone chips in the back of the elbow. While X-rays are enough for the diagnosis, we always recommend an MRI to check the status of the UCL. At times, the UCL will be significantly damaged even though it may not demonstrate symptoms at the time of presentation. Some patients will require UCL reconstruction in addition to bone spur removal.

How to Treat Bone Chips

The initial course of treatment is non-operative with activity modification, a period of rest from throwing, and anti-inflammatory medication. In this setting, a cortisone injection may be used which will decrease the inflammation surrounding loose bone chips. Pitching mechanics, where there is any inflexibility or weakness within the entire kinetic chain, need to be addressed. Patients often can return to throwing, but may have low-level symptoms. If the patient can continue throughout the season, it's reasonable to have more definitive treatment at the end of the season.

Indications for surgery include those patients who fail non-operative treatment or have maintained levels of symptoms despite being able to throw and wish to have surgery, which is commonly performed in the offseason.

Surgical technique involves arthroscopy, which uses a camera inserted into the elbow to identify the loose bone chips. A thorough examination of the elbow can be performed with the camera. The loose bodies are identified and removed with grasping instruments, and the regular bone edges can be smoothed with shaving instruments. Often, inflamed tissues such as synovium are removed. It should be noted to patients that elbow arthroscopy is technically demanding, as the elbow joint is quite small when compared to a knee or shoulder joint. The anatomy has much more complicated geometry and, finally, many nerves and vascular structures are at risk for injury.

Following surgery, the patient begins active elbow flexion extension exercises immediately. Elbow shoulder strength exercises are also initiated once swelling is reduced. Typically, six weeks after surgery, when the entire kinetic chain is strong, a throwing program is initiated.

The results of this operation are extremely predictable with regard to eliminating pain in the back of the elbow. Occasionally, patients will have continued pain because of arthritis. The greatest concern, however, is future development of collateral ligament symptoms that may require treatment. All players and patient families are, therefore, advised that, when undergoing elbow arthroscopy, there is a chance in the future of developing such symptoms.

CHAPTER 7
by John Gallucci, Jr.

FOOT AND ANKLE INJURIES: CAUSES, TREATMENTS, AND AVOIDANCE

Although injuries to the foot and ankle are not the most commonly seen injuries in baseball players, they do account for nearly a quarter of all injuries sustained in this population. In this chapter, we'll discuss some of the most commonly suffered foot and ankle injuries that regularly sideline baseball players across the world.

HOW THE ANKLE JOINT IS CONFIGURED

We need to define the bony structures of the ankle joint upfront, so we can pinpoint the position of instability. The ankle mortise is the joint made up of the distal tibia, fibula, and talus bones. Structurally, the tibia is our primary weight-bearing bone, through which ground forces are transmitted with each step. The fibula is a source of attachment for multiple ligaments, muscles, and tendons to extend from, and create action at, the foot and ankle. Seated within these two structures is the talus. The talus is a saddle-shaped bone whose primary functions are dorsi- and plantar-flexion, or the pointing and flexing of the foot.

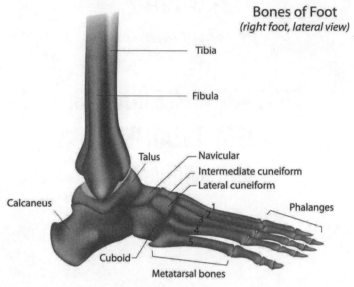

Figure 7.1

The "Tweaked" Ankle and How It Occurs

Lateral ankle sprains, when the foot rolls inward, are more common than medial ankle sprains, when the foot rolls outward. The fibula, the bone on the outside of the ankle, is longer than the tibia, the bone on the inside of the ankle, and the foot is subsequently more inclined to turn inward than outward. When the foot is pointed, the shape of the talus bone also creates an instability in which the foot is more likely to roll inward than outward. Conversely, when the ankle is flexed, it is in its most stable position. Athletic trainers will tape and brace ankles in a flexed position in an attempt to maintain as much stability as possible.

When foot and ankle injuries occur on the baseball diamond, the foot and ankle will roll, or invert, toward the midline of the body. The tendons and ligaments that maintain stability on the outside, or lateral aspect, of the foot and ankle, will overstretch, sometimes past the breaking point of their internal tensile strength.

The most commonly injured lateral ligaments are the Anterior Talofibular Ligament (ATFL), the Posterior Talofibular Ligament (PTFL), and the Calcaneofibular Ligament (CFL). All three originate from the most distal portion of the fibula, but they insert at different places: the

90

ATFL connects to the front of the talus bone at the top of the foot, the PTFL connects to the rear of the talus bone, and the CFL connects to the calcaneus, or heel bone (see Figure 7.1).

There are several classifications that cover all ligament sprains and categorize them based on the degree of the injury sustained.

DEGREES OF SPRAINS

First degree: Little fibrous tearing of the tissue. Mild swelling and pain, but joint stability is good. Most common, with a fairly short recovery period.

Second degree: Tearing of up to 50 percent. Moderate pain and associated swelling, along with moderate instability of the joint. Bulbous malleoli (prominent anklebones made up of tibia and fibula) throbbing, heat at the injury site, and difficulty walking may occur.

Third degree: More than 50 percent tissue tearing, or a complete rupture. The joint is unstable and unable to bear weight, and pain and swelling are severe. This most often occurs in the ATFL or PTFL.

HOW DOES INJURY OCCUR IN ANKLE SPRAINS?

Ankle sprains can be caused by some of the simple, daily movements involved with playing baseball. Ankles can be twisted when athletes land after catching a ball with their foot half on the base, or from sliding into a base that is raised above ground level. Ankles can be rolled from simply running on an uneven surface or falling into a divot, which can forcefully invert the ankle.

Injury risk increases based on external and environmental factors, such as playing on wet, cold, or hard turf, especially if the athlete is wearing rubber cleats.

So, I've sprained my ankle...now what?

Often, at a sanctioned athletic event, there is an onsite athletic trainer (ATC) who oversees the medical coverage for that event. This professional is capable of identifying and evaluating the extent of injury and defining a plan of care for the athlete. The athlete often needs further medical intervention, such as an X-ray or MRI, but that is up to the evaluating physician to prescribe. These tools help the medical professional see further into any minor complexities associated with the acute injury, which can range from an avulsion, in which the bone on the inside of the ankle pulls away from the ligament, to a complete fracture.

Once a physician establishes the extent of structural damage, athletes commonly seek a physical therapist for proper care and treatment of the sprain. The physical therapist is capable of treating ankle sprains of all degrees, including fractures; the reduced, or dislocated, ankle; and the postoperative ankle.

It is often necessary for the athletic trainer to immobilize the joint immediately and/or put the athlete on crutches, depending on the athlete's gait and ability to bear weight. Immobilization can be done in a walking CAM (controlled ankle motion) boot, a non-weight-bearing brace, or a cast applied by a physician. The severity of dysfunction will dictate the length of time allocated for proper healing of the various anatomical structures.

How to Treat the Acute Ankle Injury

It is important to consider the extent of damage when considering treatment and the amount of healing time associated with the diagnosis of the injured ankle. It is common to develop chronic ankle instability from improper care of, and attention to, the initial acute ankle sprain. Further damage may even be done to the bone or cartilage of the surrounding joint if a proper treatment protocol is not followed.

As always, RICE! (see Figure 4.3) Rest, ice, compression, and elevation will help to limit or decrease the initial inflammatory response. The more swollen the ankle is, the more unstable the ankle is, and the more pain you will feel. The quicker you resolve this response, the more stable the ankle will sit, and the quicker you can return to the diamond.

If properly cared for from Day One, an athlete with a first-degree sprain can typically be back to full go within two weeks, assuming there are no lingering issues of soreness or swelling. Second- and third-degree sprains will take much longer to heal, anywhere from one to six months. Injuries with further structural damage to the ligaments and/or tendons will likely have to go through a non-weight-bearing (NWB) phase and immobilization.

This will result in atrophying of the surrounding musculature: It will get weaker from a lack of use. If an athlete compares the size of the injured foot, calf, and ankle when it comes out of the boot to the uninjured side, he will often notice the injured leg is considerably smaller. For this individual, an appropriate treatment plan will include strengthening and restoration of functional movement patterns, which includes exercises to improve balance and proprioception.

SKELETAL MUSCLE PUMP – AND HOW IT HELPS TO HEAL YOU

Swelling in our bodies is sort of a necessary evil. It's our body's way of flooding an injured area with cells that assist in recovery. We need to let the body do its thing, but there are some techniques that can assist the process and limit the amount of time lost from injury.

Always, with initial trauma, our immediate goal is to limit the amount of inflammation that rushes to the area. Our bodies are great at healing themselves, and they will do just that over time, if left to their own devices. However, with less severe sprains and strains, it can be beneficial to activate what's known as our skeletal muscle pump. This process activates our lymphatic system, which is connected to our skeletal muscle, carries fluid in the body via motion, and helps pick up excess fluid. As it relates to ankle strains, a gentle flexion and extension motion of the ankle done in a "pumping" manner can help to increase lymphatic flow and decrease inflammation.

The quicker the initial swelling goes down, the quicker the athlete can advance to the next phase of the treatment protocol. Ideally, the injured ankle (or any injured joint), should be kept above the level of the heart as much as possible so gravity can assist in the process. Lying on one's back with the foot propped up (the higher the better), or on the stomach with a bent knee (ankle in the air), are both acceptable.

THE EIGHT GOALS OF REHABILITATION

There are eight goals that every physical therapist or athletic trainer set for an athlete during the rehabilitation of an injury. Completing these benchmark steps helps to ensure proper recovery and, ultimately, a return to play.

1. **Control Pain and Inflammation:** Swelling must be decreased to limit the amount of secondary cell death from the body's natural response to injury. Utilize the RICE protocol (see Figure 4.3)

2. **Restore Range of Motion (ROM):** Increase the amount of motion allowed at a joint that is otherwise limited due to injured tissue or swelling and edema. Remember, certain postsurgical guidelines specifically limit ROM for a reason, and certain benchmarks should only be reached at specific times.

3. **Restore Flexibility:** Most injury prevention protocols include programs to improve extensibility, or a muscle or muscle group's ability to be stretched, as a lack of it is often partly to blame for the injury itself and can result in secondary problems.

4. **Restore Muscular Strength and Endurance:** The health of the muscle is important for good control of an injured limb, especially a lower extremity that must bear weight. Trauma often results in muscular inhibition, or a muscle's inability to fire properly, and must be restored through therapy.

5. **Restore Balance and Proprioception:** Athletes must be able to control their limbs in often unstable environments, as well as be aware of a limb or joint's position in space. Athletes must be able to react and respond to an unstable surface while maintaining balance, control, and stability in the injured limb.

6. **Restore Cardiovascular Endurance:** It is essential for athletes to maintain as much fitness as pos-

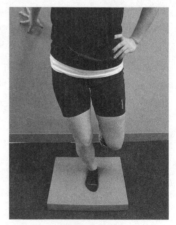

Figure 7.2

sible while away from the field. If a return to sport is expected in a short to medium time frame, including low-impact conditioning activities, such as stationary biking or swimming, along with the rehab program, is beneficial to deter deconditioning.

7. **Return to Functional Training:** To bridge the gap from the table to the field, the rehab program should include functional training activities that mimic on-field agility and reactions in a controlled

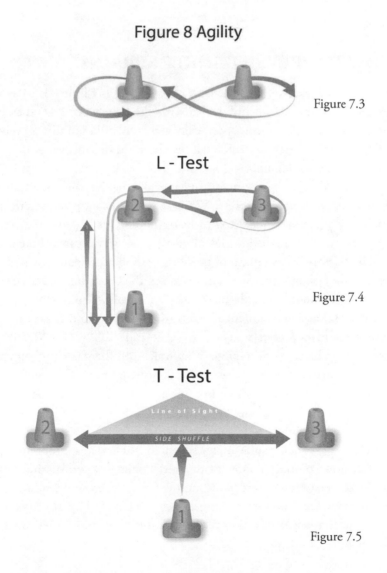

Figure 8 Agility

Figure 7.3

L - Test

Figure 7.4

T - Test

Figure 7.5

environment, such as ladder drills, figure-8 runs, and shuffling and backpedaling.

8. **Return to Sport-Specific Training:** The last step prior to a return to practice and game play is to advance to a level of training that involves any and all activities that simulate real-time game situations, but in a controlled environment. For baseball players, this should include position-specific drills, base running, and fielding balls.

HOW TO PREVENT ANKLE SPRAINS

Any ATC will tell you that the best way to treat any injury is to avoid it altogether. In this section, we will discuss the benefits of a good strength and conditioning protocol, specifically targeting ankle injury prevention. We will first begin our discussion talking about the debate over prophylactic ankle bracing and taping.

Many coaches believe ankle bracing and taping can prevent injury by assisting with ankle stability. While it is true using prophylactic ankle bracing and taping can assist with ankle stability, it is debatable whether they can prevent ankle injuries altogether. In some cases, bracing can actually decrease the strength of the surrounding musculature, which may increase the risk of injury when not wearing the brace during activity.

A lower body strength program that involves both closed kinetic chain (CKC) and open kinetic chain (OKC) exercises and targets all of the eight benchmark factors stated above is considerably more effective than prophylactic bracing and taping. Why wait until there is a problem to fix when we can avoid it altogether with a simple protocol? Of course, we are not claiming that injuries will become nonexistent, but proper strength training can dramatically decrease the risk of injury per athletic exposure.

To prevent reinjury once an athlete returns to play, it is essential to make sure the initial or acute ankle injury is treated and healed appropriately prior to a full return to sport. Following the initial trauma, secondary injuries and sprains happen much more easily, and issues can become chronic, so it is important to focus on maintaining strength and flexibility. If you continue to roll on that ankle and have yet to seek out a medical professional, it is time to do so now!

PLANTAR FASCIITIS

Plantar fasciitis results from either an acute or a chronic trauma to the bottom of the foot and occurs most commonly in those who run bases or in catchers due to the static, squatting position. Realize that this injury will keep you out of the game, and will not get better with continued activity! Treating plantar fasciitis is often difficult for athletic trainers and physical therapists because athletes are unwilling to allow for proper rest and healing.

The Anatomical Make-Up of Plantar Fasciitis

The plantar fascia is the thick band of connective tissue and associated ligaments that run along the sole of the foot, from the bottom of the heel to the base of the toes. When the plantar fascia becomes inflamed, an athlete will feel pain in the bottom of the foot, most notably in the heel.

To visualize the swelling of the plantar fascia tissue, imagine a sausage in a casing. If the casing is overstuffed, the casing will rupture. Rupturing of the plantar fascia is uncommon, but, as with the sausage, there is only so much space available within the fascial sheath, and increased swelling with continued activity causes greater discomfort and disability.

A good way to visualize the action of the plantar fascia is to think of a rubber band. Envision a proper concave arch running along the bottom of your foot. Now attach several taut rubber bands from the base of your heel to the base of each toe. Got it? Now, take your shoe off and step down on a flat surface. What happens to your foot? It splays! As the foot spreads out, the overly taut rubber bands will be stressed even more. The same thing happens to the plantar fascia when it is tight and inflamed. There is not much room for movement.

How Injury Occurs for Plantar Fasciitis

A multitude of mechanisms can cause the pain felt on the bottom of the foot. Predisposing anatomical conditions, including pes planus, or flat feet, and pes cavus, or too-high arches, are associated with plantar fasciitis.

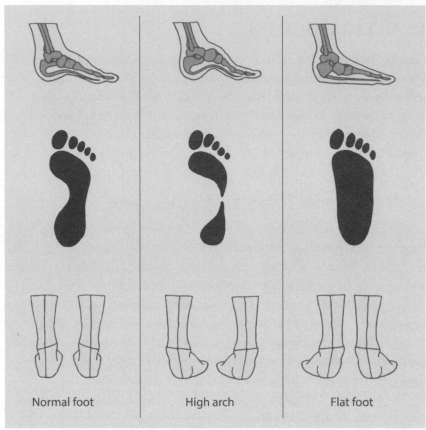

Figure 7.6

In addition to the anatomical conditions mentioned above, poor-fitting shoes and cleats can lead to improper support of the arch, ultimately leading to this painful condition. There is no one specific activity that leads to this, but it is largely related to the amount of training and conditioning performed on a weekly basis. This injury usually happens through continual running, irritating the area under the arch.

Signs and Symptoms of Plantar Fasciitis

Most initial complaints about plantar fasciitis start with how the baseball cleat feels on the foot. Athletes will say their shoe is too tight, too flat, or generally uncomfortable.

Essentially, what they're describing is an overstretching of the fascial tissue. Most commonly, after being non-weight-bearing for an extended time, for example, while sitting or sleeping, the fascia has a chance to tighten up. When we stand up and put pressure across this tissue by splaying our feet, a sharp pain is noted from the mid-foot to the heel. Pain can be reproduced with forced dorsiflexion and toe extension occurring simultaneously. This is often done during the evaluation and is a good indicator of this disorder.

The onset of plantar fasciitis can happen acutely with an overextension of the sole of the foot, but is most often progressive. As is true with any inflammatory process, the increased swelling or edema in the surrounding tissue will cause pain and tightness. This is typically exacerbated following long periods of rest. This is not an injury to which only baseball players are prone. Millions of people suffer from plantar fasciitis at some point in their lifetime.

Plantar fasciitis is exacerbated in baseball players because of the hard surfaces they train on, especially when running bases and fielding balls, as well as lengthy periods of splayed feet in catchers due to prolonged squatting and force on the arch. By limiting those variables, along with training hours, we can begin to scale back some of the damage already done. Long-standing cases of plantar fasciitis can sometimes cause a degenerative change in the tissue and lead to more inflammation that potentially causes fibrous tearing of the connective tissue of both the surrounding ligaments and tendons.

The diagnosis of plantar fasciitis is made by a medical professional through examination of the involved tissues. To properly evaluate the integrity of the medial longitudinal arch (the primary arch along the inside of your foot running from heel to toe), the patient should be barefoot, and observed in both non-weight-bearing and full-weight-bearing positions. Further evaluation may involve advanced imaging to quantify the inflammation in the fascial tissue.

How to Treat Plantar Fasciitis

The simplest approach to treating plantar fasciitis is to decrease inflammation. This can be done with prescription anti-inflammatory drugs, but, keep in mind, there will be more long-term improvement if the actual cause of the inflammation is addressed! If inflammation is severe, it may be in the best interest of the athlete to spend some time in a boot. Of course, the RICE protocol still applies (see Figure 4.3). Ice is most effectively applied to this area by giving the athlete a frozen bottle of water to roll along the sole of the foot while in a seated position.

Once the athlete becomes pain-free, flexibility of the connective tissue must be restored. The goal is to stretch the fascia, along with the heel cord and lower leg, into dorsiflexion. This will give elasticity to the entire structure and work on some of the predisposing factors.

In physical therapy and athletic training, we will use electric modalities, massage, and stretching techniques to loosen the tissue and decrease inflammation. Simple exercises are also used to strengthen the bottom of the foot, advancing to more weight-bearing or closed kinetic chain-strengthening exercises as the athlete progresses. Then, balance and proprioceptive components will be added before moving into functional and sport-specific training.

There is no quick fix for plantar fasciitis. It requires a time-consuming rehabilitation process. If the athlete does not respond to therapy, physicians may consider a corticosteroid injection to assist in the healing process. If still no progress is made, there are many surgical techniques that can be used to release the tension in the plantar fascia.

How to Prevent Plantar Fasciitis

As with every other part of the body, a proper warm-up is key. Athletes are always very concerned about loosening up their hamstrings and quadriceps, but they often forget that running athletes need their feet! The tissue at the sole of the foot needs to be kept elastic, as inelasticity leads to dysfunction. One good stretch for the plantar fascia entails wedging the foot against a wall, with the toes flexed back toward the ankle.

Inserts, both store-bought and custom-made, may be added to footwear to provide medial arch stability and help position the foot within the shoe. A medical professional can aide in the selection of such products.

For those with recurrent plantar fasciitis, night splints can help keep the fascia in a stretched position during sleep.

An athletic trainer or physical therapist can also use a technique called low-dye arch taping to support the plantar fascia in a way that mimics an orthotic or over-the-counter shoe insert.

METATARSALGIA

Metatarsalgia is a tough word to say, but it simply refers to that nagging pain at the ball of your foot. It is most often caused by…surprise… inflammation! Running and jumping athletes can develop metatarsalgia simply through overuse, but tight-fitting shoes, in conjunction with the quick acceleration and deceleration of base runners and outfielders, or the pitcher's lead foot jamming into the front of shoes, can also aggravate this condition.

The Anatomical Make-Up of Metatarsalgia

The metatarsals are the five bones that run from your mid-foot to each toe. Anatomically, the first and second metatarsals, those that correspond to the big toe and second toe, are shorter and thicker than the other three, and similar in size. During push-off, body weight is transferred to the heads of the metatarsals, and the first two absorb the majority of the force.

Mechanism of Injury for Metatarsalgia

Metatarsalgia can be an acute injury resulting from a rapid increase in running or jumping activity, or a chronic injury that develops over a long period of running and jumping.

Deviations in gait patterns and anatomical discrepancies can predispose an individual to this injury. If an athlete is coming back from another injury and is favoring one side, his or her gait may be altered. A bruise to another part of the foot can change the way an athlete strides and places his or her foot down. The ill effects of these deviations are compounded with repetitive pounding, especially in footwear that doesn't fit properly or is worn out. Other factors, such as being overweight, wearing high-heeled shoes, or having extremely high arches can contribute to metatarsalgia.

Signs and Symptoms of Metatarsalgia

Pain is most often felt at the base of toes two through four, moving from the big toe to the pinky toe. Pain increases with standing, walking, and running, but can improve when shoes are off. Some athletes describe this pain as similar to the feeling of having a rock in their shoe. Basically, the part of the foot that propels the body forward during push-off in walking and running becomes inflamed, irritated, and very sensitive.

How to Treat Metatarsalgia

Treatment for metatarsalgia targets the inflammation around the metatarsal heads. The RICE protocol (see Figure 4.3), electric stimulation, ultrasound, and LASER (Light Amplification by Stimulated Emission of Radiation) therapy can reduce inflammation. As the body reabsorbs the inflammation and the antagonist is removed, pain will begin to subside. If symptoms persist, the physical therapist or athletic trainer may elect to rest the athlete in a CAM boot, which takes pressure off the metatarsal heads at the ball of the foot.

A physician may also elect to prescribe anti-inflammatory drugs to decrease the inflammation and pain. Possibilities include ibuprofen, acetaminophen, and naproxen, which are all nonsteroidal anti-inflammatory drugs, or NSAIDs.

How to Prevent Metatarsalgia

One simple way to prevent metatarsalgia is to wear proper-fitting shoes. When recovering from metatarsalgia, it is important to not come back too soon, and to clearly, logically, and gradually progress back into activity. To prevent recurring pain, metatarsal pads, which can be found in most pharmacies, can also be used. These pads distribute the weight and force of the foot away from the metatarsal heads and cut down on the pressure occurring directly at the site of inflammation.

WHAT IS A LISFRANC FRACTURE?

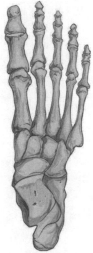

Lisfranc fractures, named for the French surgeon who first described them in the early 1800s, occur in the mid-foot, affecting the five bones that make up this portion of the foot. They allow for proper distribution of ground forces from the balls of the feet to the ankles, and, ultimately, to the rest of the body.

The Anatomical Make-Up of a Lisfranc Fracture

The foot, like the wrist, has many small bones with musculotendinous attachments that allow for greater dexterity and flexibility and provide improved motion on uneven surfaces. The Lisfranc joint complex includes the bones, tendons, and ligaments that connect the mid-foot to the forefoot, and forms the arch at the top of the foot. Ligaments and tendons in this area can be sprained, and the bones can be fractured.

Figure 7.7

The bones of the mid-foot have articulations with all five metatarsals. These bones are the three cuneiforms, the cuboid, and the navicular.

Mechanism of Injury of a Lisfranc Fracture

Direct Lisfranc injuries are the result of a trauma. They are often seen in baseball players when the athlete's foot is plantarflexed, or pointed down, and a collision occurs from an opposing player sliding into base, causing a shift in the bones. As described above, this can result in either a sprain or a fracture.

Indirect Lisfranc injuries are caused when a sudden rotational force, in positions such as a catcher, is applied to the mid-foot, whether the force is the result of contact or not. Commonly, a deformity can be seen in the foot. If not as obvious, an X-ray or CT scan should be used to look for a gap between the base of the first and second metatarsals to confirm the diagnosis.

Classifications of Lisfranc Fractures

- **Homolateral:** This describes a displacement of all bones in the same direction.
- **Isolated:** This describes a deviation of one or two bones in the same direction.
- **Divergent:** This describes the displacement of the metatarsals in varying directions.

How to Treat Lisfranc Fractures

If surgery is elected, a physician will reduce the dislocation, and may elect to pin the fracture site with an open-reduction internal fixation, or ORIF. This includes a combination of screws and wires to keep the bones and joints intact.

Recovery includes a non-weight-bearing period or a period of partial weight-bearing in a CAM walking boot. This will provide adequate time for the bone to heal, typically, six to eight weeks. Around ten to twelve weeks postsurgery, the physician will remove the screws and wiring. The athlete can then progress to weight-bearing activity, strength and balance exercises, and return-to-play activities.

It is important for the athlete to recognize that recovery will include soreness in the mid-foot, sometimes for upwards of a year, during rehab, running, and playing.

Nonsurgical treatment of a Lisfranc fracture is very similar to that of surgical rehab. Adequate time must be allowed for bone healing, either non-weight-bearing on crutches or partial weight-bearing in a boot. Then, the athlete can commence with a logical progression into weight-bearing activity, including ROM, flexibility, strength, balance and proprioceptive exercises, functional and, eventually, sport-specific conditioning.

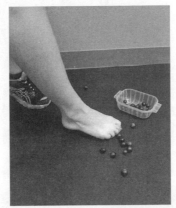

Figure 7.8

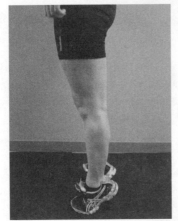 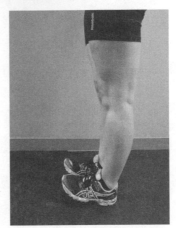

Figure 7.9

CHAPTER 8
by John Gallucci, Jr.

KNEE INJURIES : HOW THEY OCCUR AND WHAT WE DO TO TREAT THEM

The knee is one of the most complex joints in the body. It is a hinged joint that allows for minimal rotational translation—that is, side-to-side movement—and acts as a shock absorber for most athletic activities.

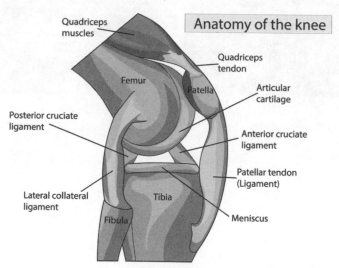

Figure 8.1

The knee joins the distal femur, or thighbone, to the proximal tibia, or shinbone. The patella, or kneecap, sits in the concave area at the bottom of the femur known as the trochlear groove.

The knee is the primary shock absorber for the lower body during the running, cutting, changes in direction, and quick stopping that occur in baseball. Just like the shocks on a car, the knee joint is subject to a lot of wear over the length of an athletic career.

A number of structures surround the knee and support and stabilize the joint. Unlike the ankle, where the bony make-up helps to support the joint when it bends up (dorsiflexion), the boniness of the knee doesn't do much to support its structural integrity. Instead, the knee has muscles, tendons, ligaments, and cartilage that maintain its stability. Muscularly, the knee is supported by the quadriceps, hamstrings, and calf; specifically, the gastrocnemius. The four main ligaments surrounding the knee are the cruciates (anterior and posterior) and collaterals (medial and lateral). The medial and lateral menisci are cartilaginous structures that cushion the knee and balance weight across the joint.

MEDIAL COLLATERAL LIGAMENT (MCL) INJURIES

The medial collateral ligament, or MCL, is located on the inner side of the knee, originating at the lower thighbone (distal femur) and inserts itself deep into the medial meniscus at the proximal tibia (the upper portion of the shinbone). It is a thick, fibrous band of tissue that is taut when the knee is extended or straightened and loses internal tension when the knee is flexed or bent. It is important to keep this in mind when considering mechanisms for spraining this structure.

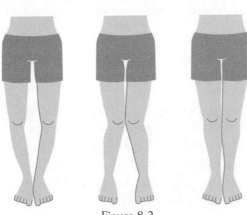
Figure 8.2

A strong valgus force, that is generated externally, is the primary mechanism for injury. Valgus force is a lateral force—that is, from the outside to the inside—that tries to force the knee beyond its normal range of motion. This often happens to an infield player who is trying to get an out when the opposing player slides into the outside of the knee, forcing it inward, or while running the bases.

As with all ligaments, there are three grades of damage, ranging in severity.

Grade 1: Few fibers are damaged. There are minor tears and some swelling—more of an overstretching than a tear.

Grade 2: There is more extensive fibrous damage, but a good portion of the ligament is still intact.

Grade 3: This is a complete, full-thickness rupture of the ligament.

Symptoms of an MCL sprain tear are an immediate onset of swelling, pain, stiffness, point tenderness over the medial joint line, and, possibly, a feeling of instability within the knee joint when walking.

It is up to medical professionals to get a full medical history, detailing exactly what happened to cause the injury, before making a diagnosis. The angle at which force was applied to the knee during injury is important. An experienced athletic trainer will be able to diagnose an MCL sprain to about 85 percent certainty based on the description provided by the athlete. Depending on the level of discomfort and disability, most sprains fall somewhere in the range between Grades 1 and 2. However, if the athlete describes hearing or feeling a "pop" to the inside of the knee, a further look via X-ray or MRI to more accurately assess the level of ligament damage is warranted. When a Grade 3 tear is suffered, the force of the injury is often such that other structures, such as the medial meniscus or ACL, can also be affected.

TREATING MCL INJURIES

A Grade 1 MCL sprain is often referred to as "the twenty-one-day injury." Within twenty-one days, the athlete should recover and be cleared for a return to sport. However, early intervention is critical to maintaining this time frame. With most Grade I and Grade II MCL sprains, it is important to treat with the RICE protocol, and physician-prescribed NSAIDs may decrease inflammation in and around the knee farther.

When returning to play, it may be helpful to use a double-hinged knee brace to help protect the MCL.

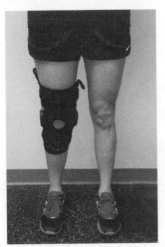

Figure 8.3

A Grade II sprain has more structural damage than a Grade I sprain and, therefore, requires a longer recovery period. As stated over and over again in this book, if athletes progress too quickly, their injuries will not heal and their pain and discomfort will continue as rehabilitation drags out. It is important for athletes to communicate with sports medicine staff as to their level of pain or any feelings of instability. If treated appropriately, athletes can expect a six- to eight-week rehabilitation prior to returning to a game.

When returning to play after a Grade II MCL strain, most athletes will describe a vibration in their knee if they return too soon. However, some pain is normal and usually goes away within a week to ten days, as long as the athlete continues with a strength and stability program.

Grade III sprains are treated very conservatively. The same benchmarks exist, but with a longer time frame allotted for the early phases of RICE, NSAIDs, and possible immobilization. The timeline may also be altered based on the athlete's degree of function. It is up to the orthopedic surgeon to determine if surgical intervention is warranted. But, regardless of the treatment decided upon, the protocol established by the medical professional will be very similar in all cases.

As always, refer to the eight goals of rehab (See Eight Goals of Rehabilitation in Chapter 7) when treating this injury.

How to Prevent MCL Injuries

MCL injuries can be prevented by following a good lower-extremity strengthening program that targets the quadriceps and hamstrings and assists the ligaments in maintaining knee stability. Also, warming up appropriately can help prepare the knee joint and the surrounding structures for action. Warm tissue is much less susceptible to injury than cold tissue.

However, due to the inherent risk in sport, and despite all precautions, injuries happen. Little can be done to completely prevent an MCL injury. However, if a baseball athlete is returning to play from a prior MCL sprain, a double-hinged knee brace can help prevent reinjury by assisting the structures that support the MCL.

ANTERIOR CRUCIATE LIGAMENT (ACL) INJURIES

Contained deep inside your knee joint are two cruciate ligaments, so defined because they cross over each other and look like the letter "X." These cruciate ligaments resist torsional (or twisting) and translational (or side-to-side) forces of the tibia on the femur.

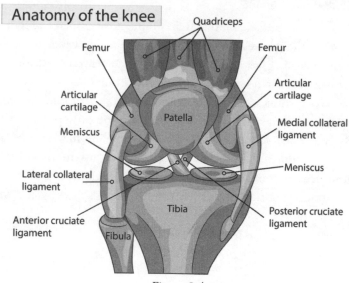

Figure 8.4

The posterior cruciate ligament, or PCL, runs from the posterior tibia to the medial femoral condyle and resists posterior tibial translation and external tibial rotation on the femur. The anterior cruciate ligament, or ACL, runs from the posterior wall of the lateral femoral condyle to the anterior tibia and resists anterior translation of the tibia on the femur and internal tibial rotation.

More simply put, the PCL resists forces that would push the tibia back in relation to the femur, while the ACL resists forces that would push it forward.

I included this long-winded explanation to detail the action that these ligaments provide in knee stabilization. These ligaments are very thick bands of fibrous tissue that provide much stability to a knee that has little else keeping it intact. They are especially important to athletes who accelerate and decelerate while running—like baseball players. Injury to these structures, especially the ACL, will cause a certain level of instability in the knee. Athletes will often describe a feeling of "buckling" when walking. It is important to note that the unstable knee is at risk for developing secondary injuries to other supporting structures, especially if athletes continue to play.

What Is the Mechanism of Injury for ACL Injuries?

There are many ways athletes can tear their ACL, but all the mechanisms of injury fall under two categories: contact and noncontact. Contact is generally used in reference to contact with an opposing athlete.

A contact injury to the ACL describes an injury in which the knee is subjected to a sudden, valgus force through contact with another person or object, such as an athlete. The force is great enough to open the knee joint to such an extent that the ACL tears. Oftentimes, we see this mechanism when a player is "rolled up on" by another player, or an opposing player falls on the back of his leg. The severity of this type of injury changes based on the tissues that are damaged. In the worst case, an athlete will suffer "the unhappy triad," which refers to a rupture of the MCL, medial meniscus, and ACL. Surgical repair is required in such an instance.

Noncontact injuries to the ACL are most often caused by a sudden twist or forceful contraction of the quadriceps with the foot planted and the knee in a valgus, or knock-kneed, position. Often, a sudden stop and change of direction, where the athlete firmly plants his or her foot in the grass or sand, is enough to stress this ligament beyond its tensile strength. Keep in mind, the tensile strength of this ligament is tremendous, but everything has its breaking point.

Signs and Symptoms of ACL Injuries

If athletic trainers are in a good position to see the mechanism of injury clearly, then 85 percent of their evaluation is already done. The job at this point is to calm the athlete and collect information. If it's determined that an ambulance is unnecessary, it is appropriate to palpate and test the knee's range of motion, possibly including a Lachman or anterior drawer test, which manually stresses the ACL to check for instability. It is best to do this test on the field right after the injury occurs because the muscles surrounding the knee will tighten up to protect the injury site. Once this muscle-guarding response happens, it is more difficult for a medical professional to diagnose an ACL tear with a physical examination.

Symptoms often described by the athlete include the feeling of a sometimes audible "pop," with immediate swelling, a feeling of instability, and difficulty bearing weight. Because this injury is so prevalent in our athletic culture, everyone tends to fear the worst. Fortunately, protocols for identifying, correcting, and restoring the athlete to prior function are on the cutting edge. The time between initial injury and full return to play has been cut down to less than one year! This, of course, assumes there was early intervention, and no difficulties arose throughout the course of rehabilitation.

How to Treat ACL Injuries

When a suspected ACL tear is sustained on the field, it is important for the athlete's knee to be immobilized and not bear weight, and, if possible, apply RICE principles to limit pain and inflammation. With a complete on-field assessment, the athletic trainer can determine the athlete's status and recommend a plan of care for further evaluation by a physician.

Depending on the circumstances—e.g., the athlete's level of pain and mobility, and the accessibility of care—it is acceptable to wait a day or two to see an orthopedist. This is not normally an injury that requires immediate medical attention, but the athlete should contact a local orthopedic surgeon right away to schedule an appointment.

Some parents prefer the peace of mind afforded by taking their child to the emergency room and getting a more immediate diagnosis. Keep in mind that many outpatient medical centers or orthopedic urgent care centers (not hospital ERs) provide the luxury of being fast-tracked to speed up the process of an orthopedic evaluation and to schedule further diagnostic testing. If the physician confirms the likelihood of knee injury, conclusive evidence can be seen through the MRI to properly define the variance of the tear, and the athlete can immediately move forward to a preoperative rehabilitation protocol to prep for surgery.

How to Repair the ACL Surgically

ACL injuries are surgically corrected about 90 percent of the time. Presurgical rehabilitation has been proven to improve postsurgical outcomes and is necessary to reduce the initial inflammatory response from trauma. Along with controlling the pain and inflammation post-trauma, the goal of the physical therapist is to restore the basic range of motion from zero to 110 degrees of flexion. Additionally, muscle activation via muscle-setting exercises helps to restore normal neurological muscle-firing patterns. Post-trauma, muscles can shut down in a neurological response known as "muscular inhibition." If the muscles cannot be fully activated, the limitation can negatively affect rehabilitation.

Most orthopedics will perform surgery fourteen to twenty-one days post-trauma to allow the body's initial inflammatory response to calm down prior to introducing the entirely new trauma that is surgical repair.

When performing ACL surgery, doctors want to replace the torn ACL with a ligament that is of similar thickness and tensile strength. Options include the autograft, which is tissue taken from the patient's own body, or the allograft, which is tissue taken from a cadaver.

The two most commonly used autograft tendons are the patellar tendon and the hamstring tendon. Because the patellar tendon has bony insertions at either end (it attaches to the patella and tibia), this graft is referred to as a "Bone-Tendon-Bone," or "BTB," graft. The bone on either end is removed and the tendon is inserted into tunnels in the femur and tibia. Only the middle third of the patellar tendon is used, leaving the outer portions of the tendon intact to allow for proper functioning of the quadriceps.

Sometimes, in running athletes or in sports that require squatting or kneeling, there can be some postsurgical knee pain at the site of excision. This area must be given time to heal and must be considered during the treatment protocol. Adequate recovery time allows the new implant to heal into the bone. The body will accept it, and the treatment protocol can progress.

The hamstring tendon is another autograft that has similar tensile strength to the ACL and yields high rates of success. This is similar to the BTB graft in every respect, except for the obvious location of excision, and the fact that it is all tendon, rather than beginning and ending with bone. Using a graft from the hamstring tendon will not affect hamstring strength in the long term.

The most commonly used allograft, or cadaver tissue, is the Achilles tendon, which is re-formed in the shape of the ACL. It is very strong and is often used based on availability. However, because cadaver tissue is a foreign substance that will be placed in the patient's body, there is a small risk that the graft will not "take" and can be rejected by the body.

All these grafts are inserted into the femur and tibia through tunnels drilled into the joint and anchored into place. It generally takes six to eight weeks for the graft to heal into the bone. During this time, the graft needs to be protected and not overstretched or damaged so stability can be restored to the knee.

It is generally agreed that those competing in athletics, or who wish to be physically active throughout their lives, need to have surgery. It is entirely up to the orthopedist and the patient to make this decision. The risk associated with not surgically repairing this ligament is secondary arthritic conditions to the joint cartilage between the femur and tibia.

Preoperative Care – What to Expect

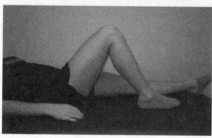

Figure 8.5

As stated previously, preoperative care is primarily designed to reduce inflammation, regain some range of motion and recover normal neuromuscular control. It is important for the physical therapist to take into account any secondary injuries that might have been sustained, whether to the meniscus or MCL, because they will often cause more pain at certain ranges of motion.

Postoperative Care – So, How Long Will This Take?

Most orthopedists are postoperatively aggressive with the ACL. Usually, the athlete will be back in rehab with a physical therapist within one to ten days of surgery. Although it may seem like a long road ahead for the athlete, the process can be broken down into stages so as not to overwhelm the athlete with timelines. In the early stages, I tell my athletes to look at their rehab as three separate, eight-week intervals. Keep in mind that, although treatment plans will be similar, orthopedic surgeons have their own postsurgical protocols. This often depends on the individual athlete and what exactly was repaired or corrected during surgery.

Phase I (Weeks 1 to 8): The most important thing during this stage is to protect the new graft! The new graft must heal into the bone, and has to be given a chance to scar down into place to restore stability in the knee. Over the course of the first eight weeks, the following should be achieved:
- Decrease pain and inflammation
- Increase ROM (Range of Motion) from 0-90 degrees
- Good vastus medialis oblique (VMO) (quad) contraction
- Manage scarring and incisions
- Progress to full weight-bearing
- Achieve a normal gait pattern

Phase II (Weeks 9 to 16): At this point, the graft has had a good chance to heal into the bone. During this eight-week period, the objective is to return joint integrity and strength, using both open and closed kinetic chain exercises. The following should be addressed:
- Work on strength of hip, foot, and ankle
- Begin leg presses
- Start functional squats
- Perform leg curls and extensions

Phase III (Weeks 17 to full RTP [Return to Play]): Every athlete enjoys this part of rehab, as they start to see the light at the end of the tunnel and can begin to return to a higher level of activity. This period should include the following:
- Running
- Directional running

- Lateral motion
- Diagonal motion
- Low-level plyometrics
- Proprioceptive and balance exercises

During these eight weeks, the athlete can also begin sport-specific activity. With the physician's permission, the athlete can begin a return-to-play protocol plan, but must realize he or she hasn't played a baseball game in six months, and return to play must be done gradually. No one wants to ruin six to twelve months of rehab by rushing back onto the diamond.

A Brief Discussion on Partial ACL Tears

Studies show that surgery is recommended to repair any fibrous tearing of the ACL greater than 50 percent of full-thickness. Of course, there are many factors that may contribute to this decision. How deep is the athlete into the season? Is the athlete returning next season? What is the athlete's current functional level? What functionality does the athlete's sport demand?

All of this must be considered in an open dialog between the athlete and the physician. The athlete must be realistic about expectations of playing at a higher level, and the athlete's safety must be taken into account. Perhaps the most important question to ask is this: What are the long-term effects of living with a partially torn ACL?

How to Prevent ACL Injuries

As the incidence of ACL injuries has increased in recent years, great programs have been developed to target the prevention of knee injuries, specifically, the ACL. Evidence-based research shows, especially with female athletes, that, with proper conditioning, we can truly decrease the incidence of ACL tears.

These programs are simple and can be applied to any athlete at any age and level of competition. Essentially, the programs teach the athlete to have proper body mechanics when jumping, landing, and rotating. While these are natural movements, a large portion of the population does not move through them properly. By retraining the body's movement patterns and decreasing vulnerabilities, injury risk can be limited to a certain extent.

Ultimately, whatever route you choose will give you the ability to decrease your risk for ACL instability. I'm of the mind-set that if you can reduce the potential loss of a season by taking an extra fifteen minutes before practice to properly warm up, why shouldn't you?

MENISCUS INJURIES: WHAT THEY ARE AND HOW TO TREAT THEM

Meniscus tears are very common in the baseball athlete and can greatly affect a player's game, if not properly cared for. This injury can affect a base runner's speed, especially while rounding the bases, a hitter's swing due to the pivot force on the knee, and cause great pain to a catcher who spends a large portion of the game in a deep squat.

The menisci act as shock absorbers within the knee joint and provide lubrication during flexion and extension of the knee. They are rubbery, cartilaginous cushions that attach to the proximal tibial plateau, which is the area within the joint that is in contact with the femur or thighbone. The meniscus is made up of two portions that are slightly different in shape. The medial meniscus is a C-shaped crescent, whereas, the lateral meniscus is more of a closed O-shape.

Proper identification of this injury can be made through evaluation, but, because the knee is a very complex joint, diagnosis can prove difficult. Most athletes will describe a catching or clicking when they bend their knee, often with intense pain associated with it. However, most athletes' knees, ankles, and hips will catch, click, and pop every day without much cause for concern. It is up to the professional to determine what is normal and what is not.

Mechanism of Injury to the Meniscus

Different mechanisms can cause meniscus tears, but they are most commonly sustained during a deep squat with a twist. With increased dynamics in this position, there is a greater risk for insult to the cartilage between the bones.

What Are the Biomechanics of the Deep Squat?

The meniscus is primarily in contact with the femur and, specifically, the femoral condyles, which are the two projections at the bottom of the femur. The condyles are thicker in front than they are in back. Biomechanically, when the knee is in full extension, the surface area is in greatest contact with the meniscus. Greater contact area means greater distribution of forces through our shock absorbers, the menisci.

Alternatively, when the knee is in a position of greater than 90 degrees of flexion, as is always seen in the deep squat, the contact area of the femoral condyles with the menisci is at its lowest. Biomechanically, less surface area in contact with the meniscus will increase the amount of force transmitted through those two points of contact.

Remember, the menisci are our primary shock absorbers in the knee. Improper wear on these structures leads to degenerative changes, resulting in pain and discomfort. While deep squats can cause degeneration, this position is often unavoidable in both athletics and everyday life, so it can be beneficial to train the body to be comfortable in that position, within reason and without excess. If it hurts, don't do it.

Signs and Symptoms of Meniscus Injuries

There are several general classifications of meniscus tears named for the way they look on radiographs: longitudinal, bucket handle, parrot beak, or mixed bundle, which is a mixture of all three. Meniscus tears present in three ways, depending on the onset of symptoms.

Acute: If an athlete feels a "pop" during a deep knee bend, he or she likely has an acute meniscus tear. Athletic trainers will probably observe swelling, joint stiffness, and an associated locking of the knee in a flexed position. The locking is often a result of actually having a flap of the torn meniscus caught in the joint, causing extreme pain at certain ranges of motion.

Sub-Acute: Sub-acute meniscus tears cause pain without affecting the functionality of the knee. They generally hurt less than acute tears. However, over time, symptoms may increase and can result in long-term pain and degeneration. If not treated appropriately, the persistent inflammation and lack of a complete meniscus can cause instability in the joint, resulting in further injury.

Chronic: Most older baseball athletes, more specifically catchers, hitters, and base runners, have some level of degeneration in their meniscus, based on a wearing or thinning over time from years of abuse. Level of pain varies with the individual. Depending on the circumstances, this player may want to consider making the transition to coaching! If degeneration is very advanced, a partial or total knee replacement may be necessary.

How to Treat Meniscus Injuries

Depending on the onset of symptoms (acute, sub-acute, or chronic), it is advised to RICE! Based on pain level and functionality, crutches might be necessary to make the joints non-weight-bearing, and NSAIDs may be used to decrease inflammation and pain.

To properly care for and treat the meniscus, it is important to understand the blood supply to the different areas of the menisci. The outside one-third of the meniscus has a rich blood supply and tears in this area, and, while often repaired with surgery, can sometimes heal on their own. In contrast, the inner two-thirds of the meniscus lacks blood supply, which means tears in this area cannot heal.

The location of a meniscus tear will often dictate whether surgery is required. If a tear occurs in an area where there is good blood supply, the body will be able to heal naturally. Without good blood supply, the tissue will simply float in the joint and continue to cause pain and discomfort. Because the body cannot heal tears in these locations, suturing the torn tissue will not provide any benefit. In this instance, it is better to just remove the torn or frayed cartilage altogether.

Surgically, meniscus tears can usually be fixed arthroscopically, with minimal invasiveness. As mentioned earlier, surgical technique to either repair or remove a section of the meniscus is dependent on the blood supply to the tissue and the location of the tear. Because meniscus tears vary, so does recovery time and rehabilitative restrictions after surgery. Surgical options are as follows:

Meniscectomy: During a meniscectomy, only the torn portion of the meniscus is removed. Length of time for full recovery and return to function is approximately six to eight weeks.

Meniscal Repair: During a meniscal repair, the surgeon will repair the torn area of the meniscus with sutures. The ability to perform a meniscal repair depends on the type of tear and its location, but also on the age and athletic level of the patient. Recovery time is four to five months and, following surgery, range of motion will be limited to 45-90 degrees of flexion within the first several weeks. The athlete will also be non-weight-bearing for four to six weeks.

Again, the postsurgical protocol is dependent on the type of procedure performed. A meniscectomy will always have a shorter recovery since there is no time frame necessary to allow torn tissue to heal back into the bone. On the other hand, a meniscal repair, where the torn portion of the meniscus is physically sutured and anchored back into the bone, needs adequate time to heal back into the bone. There is no possible way to speed this up, and more limitations are placed on the athlete postoperatively to protect the graft.

How to Prevent Meniscus Injuries

Unfortunately, there is no true way to prevent a meniscus tear. As discussed previously, studies show that strengthening the quadriceps and hamstring muscle groups to promote lower body control can increase overall stability. This can certainly reduce the risk of meniscus tears, but, once again, injury is an assumed risk in sport.

CHAPTER 9
by John Gallucci, Jr.

HIP, THIGH, AND SPINAL INJURIES

The Hip Joint

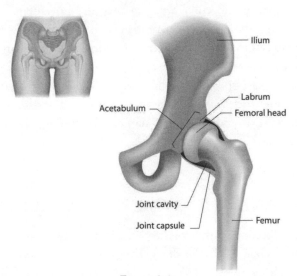

Figure 9.1

As we move even farther up the leg, we reach the hip and thigh complex. The hip joint is a ball-and-socket joint, also known as a spheroidal or multiaxial joint, in which the ball-shaped surface of one bone fits into the concave, cup-like depression of another. Unlike the knee joint, the hip joint is multidirectional and can move across all three planes of motion: sagittal, frontal, and transverse. While injuries to the upper extremity are more commonly discussed in the baseball athlete, attention must be paid to the importance of hips and legs in the throwing baseball player. Improper lower body mechanics in the throwing athlete can lead to improper upper body mechanics, resulting in less power and possible injury due to compensatory patterns.

Like all joints in the body, the hip joint contains four types of tissue that hold its structure together: bones, ligaments, muscles, and tendons. The ligaments that hold together the pelvic bones extend into the proximal femur. Because they are located deep within the musculature of the lumbo-pelvic-hip complex, or LPH, these structures are rarely injured during athletic activity. The tendons, however, transmit action from the muscles to the bone.

Approximately twenty-nine muscles make up the LPH complex, including the adductors, hamstrings, hip flexors, abdominals, erector spinae, tensor fascia latae, and gluteals. These muscles not only provide stability throughout the core, but also provide movement for walking, running, and jumping. It is important to keep in mind the close relationship that exists between the joint, the bony junctions, and the many muscles in this area as injuries are treated, prevented, and rehabilitated. As with any joint, we can isolate specific musculature for rehabilitative purposes, but we must consider the multiplanar actions of the ball-and-socket joint and their impact on surrounding joints—namely, the spino-sacral junction and the lumbar spine.

THE HIP AND THE OVERHEAD ATHLETE

When we are looking at the overhead throwing athlete and, in this case, the baseball pitcher, we break down the process of throwing a ball into six steps, which are the wind-up, early cocking, late cocking, acceleration, deceleration, and follow-through. In each of these phases, most baseball players are very familiar with the motions and injury risks that are involved in the upper extremity, but often forget that generating velocity and force behind that fastball begins in the lower half of the body. In fact, the lead foot strike that occurs at the end of the early cocking phase is what transfers kinetic energy through the legs, into the hips, core and upper body, and then, finally, into the arm, hand, and ball. Studies and injury patterns also show that forces of the shoulder and elbow are strongly related to rotation of the pelvis, and lead foot leg stride is linked to throwing velocity. With this in mind, inadequate leg stride and improper lead foot placement, whether due to poor hip strength and range of motion, pain, injury, or improper mechanics, can make quite the difference when trying to throw at top speeds.

MECHANISM OF INJURY FOR A MUSCLE STRAIN

When discussing injury to these structures, we're often referring to a strain of the musculature, which occurs when the muscle is stretched beyond its normal limit. This can result from doing too much too soon, inadequately warming up, overworking the musculature, or it can simply be caused by a chance occurrence. As with most muscular injuries, the trauma can be either acute or chronic.

An acute muscle strain results from an immediate or sudden occurrence that causes pain. Most often, this is from a rapid or violent force when the athlete is fatigued or unprepared. If it's early in the game or practice, and the athlete decides to go at it 100 percent before being properly warmed up, the muscles are not prepared for a rapid stretch-contraction. Conversely, when it's late in the game, and the athlete is dehydrated or fatigued, the muscle is also at risk for strain. So, how do we find a happy medium?

Prior to athletic activity, we need to educate our athletes on proper ways to take care of, and listen to, their bodies. A proper warm-up during which the athlete breaks a sweat means he or she is getting adequate blood into the muscles. With improved blood flow, the muscles are actively healing and increasing their extensibility, and, thus, their preparedness for activity.

Along with this, hydration is important to keep blood flowing smoothly through the various tissues. Without enough fluid intake before, during, and after activity, our blood becomes thicker and more viscous and has difficulty traveling through the body. Aside from a clear drop in performance, this also puts the athlete at a greater risk for muscle strain.

Chronic muscle strains result from the same motion repeated over and over again. The same muscles are worked relentlessly in the same muscle pattern. For this portion, let's think about kickers in American football. Their job is extremely repetitive and does not allow for much diversity in training. A kicker only kicks, but think about how much more a pitcher throws a ball.

For these athletes, it's about proper management of their practice. This is why pitchers keep a pitch count. Their time should really be spent on good, quality reps, with a strong focus on technique. It doesn't make much sense to go out and throw until their arms are ready to fall off.

Signs and Symptoms of a Muscle Strain

Signs and symptoms of a muscle strain can range from a sharp, stabbing pain during activity to a basic ache during rest. There may be swelling and, most times, there will be a visible, physical divot or spacing in the tissue. Depending on the severity or degree of the strain, you'll likely see black and blue discoloration, combined with associated pain and loss of range of motion at either the knee or hip. When looking at more true tissue tears, such as the second- and third-degree tear, an orthopedic consult is necessary.

Degrees of Muscle Tears

- **First Degree:** Overstretch of muscle fibers
- **Second Degree:** Tearing of a few fibers
- **Third Degree:** Full tear of the musculature.

It's often difficult to distinguish among the different strains without advanced imaging that can directly see and define how much tearing actually occurred. But, ultimately, the same treatment will be used regardless of degree to relieve discomfort, reduce inflammation, and protect from further damage. With any strain, it's not always necessary to immediately see a physician as long as the athlete is being properly treated. Persistent symptoms and lack of improvement within four to seven days may warrant further medical intervention.

Adductor Strain

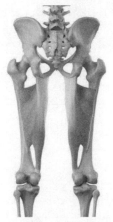

There are four adductor muscles that extend from the pubic bone to the femur: the adductor magnus, minimus, brevis, and longus. This muscle group functions to bring the leg toward or across the midline of the body.

Adductor strains occur very often, as lower extremity injuries go, in the baseball athlete, and are unique in that the area of injury has a high rate of differential diagnoses. What this means is there is a lot that could be going on in that region. So, prior to diagnosing an adductor strain, it's important to rule out other injuries, such as a sports hernia or athletic pubalgia, labral tear, hip flexor strain, or pubitis, which is inflammation between the pubic bones.

Figure 9.2

Actions that may cause pain to an athlete with an adductor strain are lifting the leg up and across the body, such as winding up to throw the ball. Keep in mind that it's not just the motion of adduction we need to limit, but also abduction of the hip that will stretch this musculature. Abduction is where you bring your leg all the way out to the side or away from the midline of the body, as seen in the lead leg when a base runner side-shuffles a few steps to get a lead off the base.

Hamstring Strain

The Hamstring Group

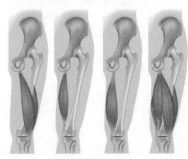

Biceps femoris   Semitendinosus   Semimembranosus

Figure 9.3

The hamstring originates at the ischium, which is the portion of the pelvic bone that we sit on. It attaches all the way down at the tibia and fibula and acts at both the hip and knee joints. It is primarily responsible for hip extension and knee flexion. There are two medial hamstring muscles, known as the semitendinosus and semimembranosus. The biceps femoris is located on the lateral side and is made up of two heads leading to a singular insertion. These large muscle bellies make up the posterior thigh musculature, with the tendons running distally, forming the borders of the space behind the knee with their corresponding tendon location. An overstretch can strain one of these three muscles acutely, with the biceps femoris being the most often strained.

Depending on the location of the damaged structures, hamstring strains are usually felt in the middle of the posterior thigh. Because the length of the hamstring muscle group covers the entire back of the thigh, you can strain this muscle in any area.

Quadriceps Strain

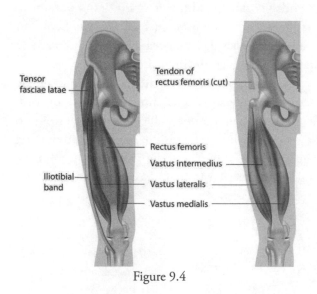

Tensor
fasciae latae

Tendon of
rectus femoris (cut)

Iliotibial
band

Rectus femoris

Vastus intermedius

Vastus lateralis

Vastus medialis

Figure 9.4

The quadriceps muscle grouping on the anterior portion of the thigh includes four powerful muscles that act to flex the hip and extend the knee: the vastus medialis, vastus lateralis, vastus intermedius, and rectus femoris. The hamstring and the quadriceps also cross two joints, acting as the primary knee extender, as well as supporting hip flexion. Of course, actions are different, but these muscles are all strained in the same manner when the muscles are stretched beyond their normal limits.

How to Treat Muscle Strains

Most baseball players try to come back from muscle strains way too quickly and do not understand the importance of rest. As discussed previously, any type of strained muscle should be treated with the RICE protocol. Instinctively, most people will try to stretch or roll out their muscle on a foam roller to alleviate their pain. This is not recommended for the acute strain! Although this can be a beneficial treatment option, it should not be performed until the muscle has had a chance to recover and heal. Before progressing into any type of functional rehab and, certainly, before returning to play, the muscle must have time to heal properly.

So when can I stretch a strained muscle?

When I see an athlete with a muscle strain, I try to decrease pain and swelling by simply using anti-inflammatory medication (NSAID), modalities, and icing. I make sure the athlete can walk without pain before progressing the rehab. Usually, the initial goals are to decrease inflammation and pain, restore normal function of the hip, and restore knee range of motion.

Sometimes, the athlete must avoid any weight-bearing with a compression bandage at the beginning of treatment. In this circumstance, it is important to understand that the muscle must heal prior to any progression to flexibility.

Once the athlete can walk, sit, and stand without pain, he or she can begin to progress into some low-level flexibility protocols. Included in this should be a strength progression beginning with muscle-setting exercises and advancing to more functional components.

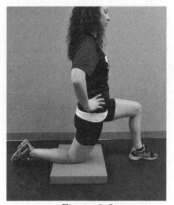

As with all rehab, it is not about just the injury, but the entire limb, taking into account the joints above and below the injury. As the patient starts to regain strength, he or she can then progress into closed kinetic-chain activities. Follow those with sport-specific activities, including plyometrics, and, ultimately, with a full return to play.

Figure 9.5

How to Prevent Muscle Strains

As with all muscular injuries, preventing muscle strains in the hip and thigh is quite simple. The muscle needs to be strong enough to handle the demands of the sport. Good training and conditioning, along with a good warm-up, are pivotal components of any athlete's fitness routine. Of course, early intervention with an injury can truly reduce the time away from the diamond. Remember that a first-degree strain can quickly turn into a second- or third-degree strain without appropriate care and attention.

Sometimes, athletic trainers will attempt what's known as a hip spica.

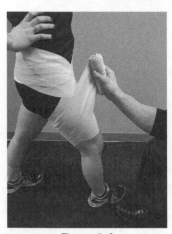

Figure 9.6

This is essentially a prophylactic bracing, where an Ace bandage is wrapped around the thigh and waist to assist the muscle action and alleviate pain. This can support a hamstring, hip flexor, or adductor strain. Depending on the injury location, positional shortening of the musculature, followed by the wrapping technique, assists the musculature during physical activity. This doesn't always work for the athlete, and it is dependent on the severity of injury, stage of return to play, and the intensity of their action as an athlete.

THE WARM-UP

As we've discussed throughout this book, the importance of a good warm-up cannot be overstated. A warm-up does not consist of a two-minute jog around the field. The purpose of the warm-up is to generate good blood flow within key musculature necessary for practice or a game and is definitively sport- and position-specific.

A good rule of thumb is that the athlete should be sweating prior to engaging in athletic activity. Depending on the athlete's sport and position, some musculature is used more often than others.

MUSCLE CONTUSION

A muscle contusion, or bruise, is the result of direct impact to the muscle. Baseball athletes most often suffer a contusion when a baseball hits them directly over a muscle. The direct blow will likely cause broken blood vessels and subcutaneous bleeding. Once this happens, blood will pool in the area. Although most often mild, muscle contusions can be quite painful and, if not treated properly, can actually result in a calcification of the muscle known as myositis ossificans.

Myositis ossificans can be explained by looking at its name: the muscle (myo) ossifies, or forms bone, resulting in a lack of mobility and flexibility within the muscle group. To properly treat this, we have to instill a protocol of RICE and flexibility! The athletic trainer or physical therapist may want to use electrical stimulation to control pain, as well, but the most important components at play here are icing to decrease the blood pooling in the area and stretching to maintain muscle flexibility.

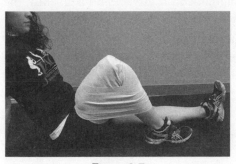

Figure 9.7

There are two things we never want to do when treating myositis ossificans. First, we don't want a second impact to be suffered during play, so proper padding is required. Second, we don't want to apply moist heat as we often do with muscular injuries. With any acute trauma, the body will initiate its own inflammatory response, bringing fluid to the area. Moist heat only increases the fluid volume and hastens cellular death, while icing and stretching combat those symptoms.

As stated above, these cases are usually mild, but can be classified more severely based on the symptoms of pain, swelling, stiffness, and loss of function.

LABRUM TEARS

The hip joint is another ball-and-socket joint with articulations between the femur and pelvis, with the femoral head being the ball, and the pelvis the socket. This allows for a larger range of motion at our hips. The labrum is a layer of cartilage at the articular surface of the pelvis that provides added stability to the femoral head as it sits in this groove. The labrum also provides a smooth surface for the bones to glide against one another.

Much of the actual stability at the hip joint is provided by the massive amount of musculature in the area. Many muscles, including the glutes, hamstrings, quadriceps, psoas, tensor fascia latae, and many other small rotators originate at the pelvis and attach at the femur. Remember, there are twenty-nine individual muscles that make up your lumbo-pelvic-hip complex! So, while there is tremendous range of motion at the hip, there is also a lot holding it in place.

A final important detail to consider in this joint is the shape and orientation of the femoral neck and head. Although this ball-and-socket joint is similar to your shoulder in many ways, a major difference is the femoral neck as it angles into the pelvis. The orientation can vary in all three planes of motion: frontal, sagittal, and transverse. Subsequently, the femoral head can have various dynamics as it articulates with the pelvis. Depending on the mechanics of the insertion of the femoral head, as well as its shape (no one's is perfectly round like an actual ball!), some people have a higher risk for injury to the labrum or surrounding structures.

MECHANISM OF INJURY FOR LABRUM TEARS

As with most injuries we've discussed thus far, there is a difference in the acute versus chronic mechanism of labral tears.

Acute labral tears most often occur with a dislocated or subluxated hip. A subluxation is a dislocation with a rapid, spontaneous reduction. That is, the hip pops out and then goes back in. Although rare, due to the large amount of musculature holding the hip joint in place, this injury results from a violent force with high velocity, and can create trauma not only to the labrum, but to the surrounding structures, as well. Please note that a hip dislocation is a medical emergency, and should be treated as such, because the blood supply to the lower limb can be compromised. The possibility of an occluded or obstructed artery supplying the leg is very real, and must be treated with care. Never should anyone attempt to relocate or reduce a hip dislocation on the field. This should be done under the care of a physician at a trauma center, where proper equipment is available.

The trauma of the femur sliding out of its natural articulation with the hip socket may tear the labrum. A true diagnosis of a labrum tear is confirmed with an MRI arthrogram, where dye is injected into the hip for an accurate depiction of the joint structures, which are difficult to discern on a regular MRI. A radiologist will confirm the diagnosis from the images taken and determine the degree of tear ranging in severity from a mild Grade 1 to a most-problematic Grade 4.

Chronic labral tears are caused by repeated insult to the labrum. This can be the result of an anatomical deformity or abnormality in the way the femoral head is shaped, or how it articulates with the hip socket, which causes unusual wear and tear on the joint cartilage. For baseball athletes, forceful twisting, rotation, flexion, and extension of the hip on a daily basis are unavoidable. It may not stop us from playing, but it can cause degeneration of the labrum.

Signs and Symptoms of Labral Tears

Most often, a labrum tear will present to an athletic trainer as anterior hip pain. Because there are a number of tissues in the area that could be the source of the pain, it is always important to rule out any intra-articular hip pathology prior to confirming any other diagnosis. In this instance, the labrum is the intra-articular hip pathology we most often look for. Athletes will present with painful ranges of motion, possibly describing a click or a catch in the groin that comes and goes. Groin strains can often be misdiagnosed as a labrum tear, and a labrum tear can often be misdiagnosed as a groin strain. An MRI arthrogram is necessary for a proper diagnosis.

How to Treat Labral Tears

Initially, athletic trainers and physical therapists often treat labrum tears conservatively, first using the RICE protocol to limit inflammation. Due to the multiple muscular attachments in the area and the possibility of tight musculature leading to pain, manual therapy techniques can often be helpful in treating less severe cases. Unfortunately, with a labrum tear, there are only so many treatment techniques and options available in a rehabilitation setting. Ultimately, it comes down to the athlete's level of discomfort and ability to compete at a high level. The labrum cannot heal itself, but pain can be managed in a variety of ways, including NSAIDs and steroid injections.

As pain is always the best subjective guideline, if pain persists, and treatment no longer yields improvements, it is time for athletes to follow up with a physician to see what their options are moving forward.

Surgical Intervention

If conservative treatment options have been exhausted, surgical intervention may be necessary. Depending on the cause and extent of the labral tear, the surgeon can either excise, or remove, the torn piece of labrum, or repair the torn tissue by sewing it back together. Depending on the anatomy and mechanism of injury, there may be different tweaks to the procedure to reduce the risk of recurrence. Such things might involve shaving down an abnormal extension of the femur that is destroying the cartilage.

However the surgeon decides to repair the joint, a specific treatment plan will be detailed to protect the acutely repaired hip. Following surgery, it can be upwards of six months before the athlete is ready to return to the diamond, but there is a good success rate with labral repair surgery.

How to Prevent Labral Tears

Labral tears are prevented by good strength, flexibility, and balance components in a training regimen. Making sure athletes have equal strength and control on both sides of their bodies is key. Doing the right stretches to keep the hips flexible and mobile is also beneficial. As with any injury, early intervention often helps to limit or deter insult to tissue.

LUMBAR SPINE INJURIES

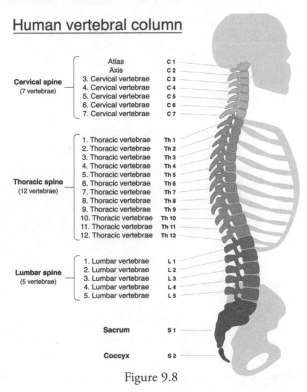

Human vertebral column

Cervical spine (7 vertebrae)	Atlas	C 1
	Axis	C 2
	3. Cervical vertebrae	C 3
	4. Cervical vertebrae	C 4
	5. Cervical vertebrae	C 5
	6. Cervical vertebrae	C 6
	7. Cervical vertebrae	C 7
Thoracic spine (12 vertebrae)	1. Thoracic vertebrae	Th 1
	2. Thoracic vertebrae	Th 2
	3. Thoracic vertebrae	Th 3
	4. Thoracic vertebrae	Th 4
	5. Thoracic vertebrae	Th 5
	6. Thoracic vertebrae	Th 6
	7. Thoracic vertebrae	Th 7
	8. Thoracic vertebrae	Th 8
	9. Thoracic vertebrae	Th 9
	10. Thoracic vertebrae	Th 10
	11. Thoracic vertebrae	Th 11
	12. Thoracic vertebrae	Th 12
Lumbar spine (5 vertebrae)	1. Lumbar vertebrae	L 1
	2. Lumbar vertebrae	L 2
	3. Lumbar vertebrae	L 3
	4. Lumbar vertebrae	L 4
	5. Lumbar vertebrae	L 5
	Sacrum	S 1
	Coccyx	S 2

Figure 9.8

Whether they are baseball players or not, thousands of Americans suffer from lower back injuries. In a normal, healthy individual, the lumbar spine curves in an anterior to posterior direction. If you look at the lumbar spine from the side, the curve is slightly concave. Because the human body likes to be in balance, if there is a sway too far in one direction, there is always a corrective sway in the opposing direction. This gives us balance in our upright posture and allows us improved functionality throughout our daily activities.

However, excess curvature in the spine can lead to kyphotic or lordodic curvature. Lordosis, or swayback, is a condition in which the spine in the lower back is excessively curved, putting extra pressure on the spine and causing pain. Kyphosis is an exaggerated rounding of the upper back, sometimes referred to as a hunchback.

Certain body types are more prone to an exacerbation of the curvature of the spine, or, conversely, a lack thereof, causing problems above and below that area of the spine.

Lumbar Strains

Baseball athletes place a large amount of torque, or rotational force, upon their lower back at very quick speed while hitting and pitching, for example. This stresses the lower back's musculature and bony processes. They also commonly use one side of their body more often than the other, and that repetitive overuse on a single side of the body often leads to weakness on the opposite side. For a variety of reasons, baseball players often suffer lumbar strains (see muscle strain explanation above) to the muscles that run along both sides of the spine. Lumbar strains often result in lower back spasms.

The pain caused by a lumbar strain comes on quickly and can be accompanied by loss of motion or strength, and an inability to flex, extend, and rotate the trunk.

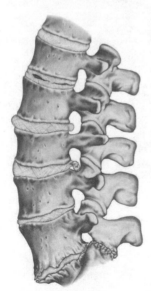

Figure 9.9

Lower back spasms are generally the result of the spinal vertebrae being out of position. While back pain can sometimes be caused by problems in the back, it is more often the result of a dysfunction in the structures that attach directly to the lumbar spine and pelvis. It is important to determine the actual cause of the back pain and treat it directly.

Hamstring Group

The hamstring muscles attach to the inferior portion of the pelvis and, due to their location on the posterior, tend to pull in that direction. An athlete with "tight hamstrings" will have difficulties with the entire posterior chain. This athlete will often present with a "flat back," which occurs when the hamstrings are so tight they pull the pelvis backwards, flattening out the normal curve in the lower back. This leads to a weakening of the quadriceps and back muscles and may cause back pain.

Quadriceps/Hip Flexor Group

The quadriceps and hip flexors attach directly to the anterior pelvis and lumbar spine. Tightness in this muscle grouping will lead to an anterior pull on the pelvis and an increased lordotic curve, which can also cause back pain.

How to Treat Lumbar Strains

Once you have determined that you are dealing with a lumbar strain, the first step of treatment is the RICE protocol, as seen in Figure 4.3. I suggest a consult with a physician to rule out any type of herniation or spondylolysis, or a stress fracture of the vertebrae.

It is also important to test for any radiculopathy that may be present so more serious injury can be ruled out. If there is no radiculopathy, we can assume the pain is local and, most likely, the result of a strain or sprain. A physical therapist or athletic trainer can easily rehabilitate this with the use of modalities, and by increasing flexibility of the hamstrings, quadriceps, glutes, and paraspinal muscles, which run parallel to, and support, the spine. In addition to a flexibility program, good core strengthening can also treat and prevent lower back pain.

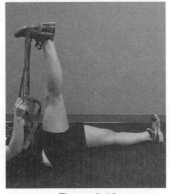

Figure 9.10

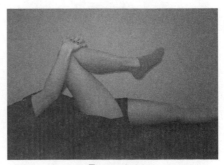

Figure 9.11

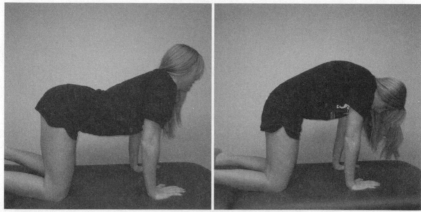

Figure 9.12

These same exercises can be used in a prevention program to reduce the risk of injury. Other ways to prevent lower back spasms are to incorporate a good warm-up prior to activity and cool down after activity that includes a flexibility routine to target problem areas. If the hamstrings or quads are tight, stretch them.

It is also important that the athlete understand the concept of core strengthening, which will be further detailed in Chapter 12 (strength and conditioning chapter).

Disc Herniations of the Lumbar Spine

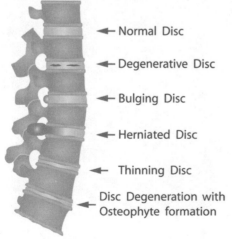

←— Normal Disc

←— Degenerative Disc

←— Bulging Disc

←— Herniated Disc

←— Thinning Disc

←— Disc Degeneration with Osteophyte formation

More aggressive lumbar injuries that can affect baseball players include the herniation, or bulging, of the inter-vertebral disc. Discs are often likened to jelly donuts: Each one is made up of an outer band called the annulus fibrosus that surrounds a gel-like substance called the nucleus pulposus. When a disc is herniated, the outer band is cracked or broken, and the gel inside the disc leaks through into the spinal canal and can place pressure on the spinal cord.

The most common disc herniations happen at level L4-L5, where the L5 nerve root is pinched, and at level L5-S1, where the S1 nerve root is pinched. An L5 nerve impingement causes weakness that extends all the way to the big toe, and can cause numbness and pain on the top of the foot and pain in the buttocks. An S1 nerve impingement causes ankle reflex and weakness during ankle push-off when running and walking. Numbness and radiating pain may extend all the way down to the bottom of the foot, as well as into the associated muscles.

Four Stages of Disc Herniation

- **Disc Degeneration:** Chemical changes, often associated with age, cause the discs to weaken but not protrude.
- **Prolapse:** The shape or position of the disc changes and creates a slight impingement into the spinal canal; also called a protrusion or a bulging disc.
- **Extrusion:** The gel-like nucleus pulposus breaks through the wall of the disc but remains within the disc.
- **Sequestration:** The nucleus pulposus breaks through the wall of the disc and spills into the spinal canal.

How to Treat Disc Herniations of the Lumbar Spine

As with any disc herniation, the athlete should immediately be under the care of both a physician and a physical therapist or athletic trainer to determine a progression of care. The goal is to decrease any present radiculopathy and try to isolate the pain locally to the lumber region. This can be done with RICE, anti-inflammatory medication, and modalities. Once radiating symptoms and pain have subsided, the baseball player can start a flexibility and strengthening program to maintain restored posture.

Herniations can also be treated with sets of exercises designed to resolve any radicular symptoms in the legs and localize pain to the lower back. Once symptoms begin to subside, either of these systems is a great tool for the beginning of rehabilitation. Once flexibility and range of motion have increased, the athlete can begin a core stabilization program, followed by a return to a functional sport routine. Once he or she has completed all these phases in a pain-free manner, the athlete may safely return to play.

Depending on the severity of dysfunction, the physician may elect to administer an epidural, a steroid injection, or even to intervene surgically. It is important to treat any radicular symptoms right away to prevent the long-term effects of nerve-root impingement, such as weakness and disability.

Spondylolysis

Due to the repetitive, powerful, high-velocity rotational forces that are required in hitting and throwing, we are seeing a large number of spondylolysis cases in our youth athletes. Spondylolysis is diagnosed when a stress fracture develops on a portion of the vertebrae called the pars interarticularis, which also happens to be the weakest spot on the vertebrae. This condition typically occurs in the lower back at the lumbar vertebrae L4 or L5 and can occur on one or both sides. Spondylolysis, if left untreated, can advance to spondylolisthesis, which is when the affected vertebrae slips forward relative to the vertebrae below.

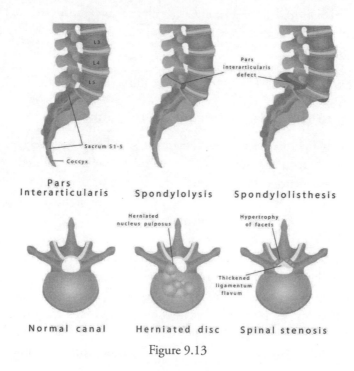

Figure 9.13

Spondylolysis can sometimes be tricky to detect as it oftentimes can initially present with no pain or very moderate pain, and the location of the stress fracture occurs on the opposite side of the aggravating activity. For example, the fracture site on a lefty pitcher would be on the right side. Athletes who do experience symptoms often complain of lower back pain presenting on one or both sides, back and hamstring tightness, point tenderness over the affected lumbar vertebrae, and pain following activities that require back extension, or bending the spine backward.

How to Treat Spondylolysis of the Lumbar Spine

The majority of spondylolysis cases can be successfully treated conservatively if the defect is detected and treated early on. Conservative management of this injury involves rest and removal from sports and other activities that aggravate the condition. Once the pain ceases, a physical therapy program that focuses on lower extremity flexibility, especially in the hamstrings, and core and trunk strengthening, is recommended. After completing the physical therapy program, the athlete may slowly return to sport-specific activities such as throwing and hitting. When the athlete is released for a full return, parents should modify the athlete's amount of playing time. For instance, athletes who typically play on three or four teams in three out of the four seasons may be wise to limit themselves to one season and one team in their first year back.

How to Prevent Disc Herniations and Spondylolysis of the Lumbar Spine

As mentioned repeatedly in this book, the rotational forces placed upon the athlete's hips and lower back cannot be prevented on the baseball diamond, and these forces, unfortunately, sometimes cause herniated disks. However, if the baseball player is well conditioned and practices proper body mechanics, he or she greatly reduces the risk of injury. The entire body must be trained to endure the demands of the sport. It is important to train both sides of the body equally, using both strength and flexibility components.

CHAPTER 10
by John Gallucci, Jr.

CONCUSSIONS: DANGERS, SYMPTOMS, AND TREATMENT

The most common head injury, not only in baseball, but in sports today, is the concussion. Parents, coaches, and players all need to recognize that a concussion is not like any other injury. It is a traumatic brain injury that can have lasting effects and can potentially be harmful to daily living by affecting the way we think, feel, and move. Unlike the upper and lower extremities, we have only one brain and, if the brain is injured in any capacity, we can also assume cognitive dysfunction will be injured on some level, with a possible loss of function that can be temporary or permanent.

As the rate of concussion increases in professional sports, and more research is done about the lasting effects, the injury is being increasingly discussed, both in the medical community and among the general public. Professional sports leagues in the United States have spent millions of dollars investigating the true causes of concussion, along with its lasting effects and treatment, and the treatment of post-concussion syndrome. We have learned that concussions do not only affect the body and how a person physically feels; they also affect speech, vision, balance, long- and short-term memory, and can be detrimental to the neurological, psychological, and cognitive well-being of the individual.

With four to five million concussions documented yearly in the United States, it is safe to assume that every player, parent, or coach has either experienced a concussion firsthand or knows someone who has. And, if they haven't, it is unlikely that any player, parent, or coach has not heard about the concussion issue. Its recent exposure in the media has alerted the public to the dangers of this trauma and the proper procedural steps to take in the event of injury.

MECHANISM OF INJURY

A concussion is caused by a trauma to the head, which is any force, either direct or indirect, that brings concussive energy to the brain.

<u>Direct Trauma</u>

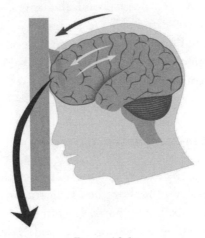

Figure 10.1

A direct trauma is most obviously caused from a blow to the head that creates enough momentum to cause the brain to slide back and forth against the inner walls of the skull. Although the skull is the brain's primary line of defense against the outside world, the trauma that causes a concussion is actually the result of the brain bouncing off the inside of the skull. Direct trauma can also cause rotational or torsional force of the cranium around its spinal axis. Such rotational forces often result in more severe concussion symptoms.

Indirect Trauma

The increased knowledge of concussions throughout the world teaches us that concussions don't only result from direct blows to the head. Concussions are the result of the velocity of the brain within the skull. Any action that causes accelerated or decelerated forces can cause a sudden shift of the brain. Imagine a baseball athlete who takes a spill backwards and falls on his backside. Force from the hard ground is transmitted up the spine and directly to the cranium, providing the necessary force to cause concussive trauma. This can be caused by any action that creates a whiplash-like, jerking motion of the head. When such motion takes place, the brain undergoes immediate biochemical changes. The normal activity of neurotransmitters—the molecules that carry signals from neuron to neuron—is disrupted. Blood flow to the brain is decreased, and the ability of neurons to use glucose as fuel is impaired. All these issues can cause global brain dysfunction.

CAN A CONCUSSION BE PREVENTED?

As athletic trainers, we are always of the mind-set that the best way to treat an injury is to prevent it altogether. Unfortunately, there are certain assumed risks of participating in sports. Despite these risks, we are always discovering and reinventing our best-practice models to align with the most current research.

As an athletic trainer/physical therapist dealing with baseball players for the past twenty-five years, I have seen different helmets, padding, and headgear targeted at preventing concussions. We can try using headgear to soften the external blow, but, in my opinion, there is really no helmet or additional padding that can act to prevent the internal impact of a concussion.

SIGNS AND SYMPTOMS OF CONCUSSION

All baseball players, coaches, and parents need to have a general understanding of the common signs and symptoms of a concussion.

To determine the severity of trauma, medical professionals rely on observational data (what can be seen and observed) as well as subjective data (what the athlete describes). Each athlete is an individual and, more so with concussions than any other injury, the expressed signs and symptoms are going to vary from person to person.

An important fact to keep in mind is that symptom onset can be immediate or delayed by days, or even weeks. Athletes with potential brain trauma must be evaluated immediately and must continue to be evaluated.

Please note that there *does not* need to be a loss of consciousness for a concussion to occur. This injury is very specific to the individual, and some people with a lower injury threshold are simply more susceptible than others.

The most common symptoms of concussion include, but are not limited to, the following:

- Headache
- Nausea
- Vomiting
- Dizziness
- Fogginess
- Confusion
- Balance Problems
- Difficulty Concentrating

Other signs and symptoms can vary over time and can include sensitivity to light and/or noise, difficulty in concentrating on TV, schoolwork, or in conversation, changes in mood, anxiety, depression, sleep disturbances (sleeping more or less), and difficulty sleeping through the night.

As a practitioner, I can tell you that these injuries are rarely clear-cut. Signs and symptoms are never the same, they don't always appear right away, and there's no timeline on a definitive resolution. We must reevaluate daily to track the progression of symptoms. As stated above, all we truly have is observational and subjective data to rely on. There are other tools we can use to frame the injury, such as computer programs that define reaction times, memory, and delayed recall, but not all athletes will have access to such diagnostic testing.

HOW TO TREAT CONCUSSIONS

An athlete suspected of having a head injury needs to be removed from participation immediately and remain shut down until properly evaluated by a medical professional trained in concussion management. I cannot stress this enough! If there is even a questionable head trauma, the risks of continued participation are too great to continue playing.

As a health-care professional practicing at all levels of competition, I have had the distinct benefit of seeing programs develop over the years and have assessed the practicality of various treatment modules.

The best-practice approach, outlined below, has evolved over the years and is now trickling down from the professional leagues to collegiate and high school athletics.

If concussion symptoms do not resolve within two to three weeks, it may be beneficial to see a neuropsychologist for proper evaluation. Because it may be required later on, it is important to document the course of symptoms from the date of injury, as well as any pre- or post-injury testing.

There are numerous neurocognitive tests available that extract data useful in diagnosing and defining this tricky injury. For example, the SCAT3 Sport Concussion Assessment Tool is readily downloadable on the Internet for public use and asks questions that establish cognitive, balance, and coordination baselines for each athlete. In the best-practices model, the athlete will take a baseline test during a pre-participation exam. He or she will then immediately follow with a post-injury exam, and again once symptoms begin to resolve, so all the exams can be compared to assess cognitive function.

When rehabilitating concussions, it is very important that the physician, baseball player, parents, and coaches are all communicating to make sure everyone is on the same page and there are clearly defined objectives.

Once symptoms have resolved and a physician trained in the evaluation and management of concussions has cleared the athlete, he or she may begin a return-to-play protocol under the guidance of an athletic trainer or physical therapist. This physical return-to-play protocol consists of six stages, with at least twenty-four hours in between each stage, which must be successfully completed sequentially to return to play. Successful completion of a stage is defined as going through the defined protocol asymptomatically. If symptoms recur during any of the stages, the athlete must rest until the symptoms resolve and then resume the program, beginning on the previous asymptomatic stage.

PHYSICAL POST-CONCUSSION RETURN-TO-PLAY PROTOCOL

Stage 1: No activity. Physical and cognitive rest. Minimum one week removal from all exertional activities. Possible removal from school. After a full week of being symptom-free, progress to Stage 2.

Objective: Allow for complete resolution of symptoms prior to introducing physical or cognitive stress that may exacerbate symptoms.

Stage 2: Introduction of light aerobic exercise at less than 70 percent of maximum heart rate on an arc trainer, stationary bike, or elliptical machine. Conditioning must be low-impact to prevent jarring to the cranium. Duration should be between fifteen and twenty minutes, depending on the athlete's prior conditioning level, which is dependent on the athlete's sport and activity level.

Objective: Introduction of mild aerobic stress. Often, when returning from concussion, symptoms may emerge with an increase in blood pressure. The residing ATC or PT will monitor the program and evaluate the athlete's progress. Note: Max heart rate is calculated using the formula "220 - age." Multiply this by 0.70 to reach the target of 70 percent. Example: 70 percent of maximum heart rate for a fifteen-year-old athlete is 140 bpm.

Stage 3: Introduction of low-impact activities. Begin with a warm-up on the bike or elliptical and progress to body-weight exercises such as lunges and squats, then to a light jog. Introduce light shuffling, cutting, and ladder drills.

Objective: Maintain the same level of intensity as Stage 2, but increase the length of time from twenty to sixty minutes, mimicking the demands of the athlete's sport.

Stage 4: Incorporate noncontact, sport-specific drills. Conditioning intensity can be increased up to 90 percent of the maximum heart rate and include sprinting, running, and cutting drills. Progressive resistance exercises with stretch and strength bands can also be introduced. Base running and a game of catch can be added.

Objective: To continue to be symptom-free as activity level increases. Upon successful completion, the athlete should be reevaluated by a physician trained in the management of concussions.

Stage 5: Return to practice. Day 1 at 50 percent, participating in half of the reps as the rest of the team. No contact or collision. The athlete can progress to a full practice as long as symptoms do not recur. Continue with cardio and strength training. The athlete must achieve his or her prior level of conditioning before returning to any baseball game.

Objective: To stress the athlete in as close to full-participation as possible without the risk of reinjury or the return of symptoms.

Stage 6: Symptom-free. The athlete is basically back to normal. Full medical clearance from a physician trained in the management of concussions is given. The athlete can then participate in a full-contact baseball practice.

Objective: Acclimatize the athlete back into team sport. This stage is necessary, mostly as a confidence builder, and must be achieved before a baseball player may reenter the game.

Returning to sport post-concussion is a delicate process. This is a vague injury, with various symptoms that may or may not be present and that may develop over time. With such an open-ended description of details, there is just as open-ended a return-to-play protocol. There is much room for interpretation, and even creativity, on the practitioner's part. As general objectives are defined, guidelines are followed, and common sense is practiced, the athlete can have a safe and healthy return to sport.

The length of the return-to-sport protocol following concussion often frustrates athletes, parents, and coaches who sometimes feel medical professionals are being overbearing or too careful. This may be true, but the risks involved are too great to ignore and, due to the potentially damaging effects of concussion, it is much safer to err on the side of caution. Further, this protocol allows for a logical, graded progression back into sport. All is evidence-based, and the goal of the medical professional is to safely prepare and return the athlete to the field. Of course, if an athlete does not adequately complete a stage of rehabilitation, he or she may be held back, which is why sticking to the program is important.

RETURN TO COGNITION IS EQUALLY IMPORTANT

In addition to reacquiring the physical skills and conditioning needed for a return to sport, the athlete must also recover cognitively. For the student-athlete, it is important to include teachers and guidance counselors in the conversation so necessary accommodations can be made. The athlete should be aware that any cognitive stressors may delay recovery and/or exacerbate symptoms. These include reading, television, video games, and texting, all of which require brain function (at least on some level!). So, don't forget, though mild, a concussion is a brain injury.

The stages of cognitive return-to-function include modifications for gradual reintegration into a full day of class or work. Similar to our physical return-to-play protocol, each stage needs to be completed in succession. If, during any stage, the athlete exhibits any return of concussion symptoms, or the onset of new symptoms, he or she should be pulled back from the current level of cognitive activity. Following twenty-four hours of rest, he or she may continue progressing through the program.

Based on new concussion research, an overwhelming majority of states have actually passed legislation on concussion safety that details proper treatment protocols. Most of those that have not yet passed legislation are in the process of doing so.

Stages for Cognitive Return to Function

STAGE	ACTIVITY	OBJECTIVE
No activity	Complete cognitive rest – no school, homework, reading, texting, video games, or computer	Recovery and resolution of symptoms.
Gradual re-introduction of cognitive activity	Remove above restrictions for short periods of time; 5-15 minutes	Gradual increase in sub-symptom threshold cognitive activities
Homework at home before school work at school	Homework in longer increments (20-30 minutes at time)	Increase cognitive stamina by repetition of short periods of cognitive activity
School re-entry	Part day of school after tolerating 1-2 cumulative hours of homework at home	Re-entry into school with accommodations
Gradual reintegration into school	Increase to full day of school	Accommodations decrease as cognitive stamina improves
Resumption of full cognitive workload	Introduce testing, catch up with essential work	Full return to school; may commence return-to-play protocols

(Source: The Buffalo Concussion Clinic)

RECURRENT CONCUSSIONS

It is important to note that repeated concussions may lower an athlete's "concussion threshold." That is, the force of impact required to produce concussive symptoms will be lower than it was prior to the athlete's first concussion. Repeated concussions can also lead to more severe and longer-lasting symptoms with each successive injury. This is why it is important to know how many concussions an athlete has had over the course of his or her season or career. As a general rule, any athlete who suffers three concussions in one season should be done for the season and examined by a neurologist.

WHAT IS CTE (CHRONIC TRAUMATIC ENCEPHALOPATHY)?

Recent headlines feature more and more retired athletes from the NFL with troubling outcomes following successful careers. It is believed by most medical professionals that, through years of traumatic abuse to the brain due to the rigors of their sport, a buildup of tau protein develops around brain tissue causing a condition called Chronic Traumatic Encephalopathy. This protein has a chemical effect on the brain and negatively affects its function. Up until recently, accurate diagnosis could only be obtained through an autopsy. However, recent developments in MRI detect the presence of this protein in living patients.

CTE is certainly not exclusive to retired NFL players. This has been seen historically in boxing, and is often described as being "punch-drunk." Symptoms include chronic headaches, depression, difficulty concentrating, memory problems, personality and emotional changes, Parkinson's, and even early onset Alzheimer's. CTE has also been found in military veterans coming back from battle who were exposed to concussive forces. As it is currently understood, CTE develops after years of repeated, sub-concussive forces. That is: forces that jar the brain but are not necessarily significant enough to cause a concussion.

CHAPTER 11
by John Gallucci, Jr.

HYDRATION AND NUTRITION FOR THE BASEBALL ATHLETE

Athletes often forget that injuries can be prevented through proper nutrition and hydration. Yes! If athletes eat and drink to properly fuel their bodies, they will stay healthier!

Baseball athletes should have a good understanding of what it means to fuel their bodies in preparation for the physical demands of their sport, as well as what foods to stay away from. For example, baseball is not a game of continuous cardiovascular activity like soccer or ice hockey, so baseball players do not need to consume extra calories, but the warmer weather of their season makes remaining hydrated critically important.

HYDRATION

Hydrate or die. That's the truth. In baseball, the ramifications of improper hydration due to the warmer weather can pose numerous potential illnesses and injuries, such as heat exhaustion, heatstroke, and muscular cramping. Baseball athletes must understand what it means to be properly hydrated, when to hydrate, and how hydration aids in injury prevention.

Sixty percent of our entire body mass and 90 percent of our blood is made up of water! Our bodies crave water, and we have to give our bodies what they want, especially during training and activity in warmer weather climates. Physiologically, water assists the human body in almost every function. It keeps the vital organs working properly, lubricates the joints, maintains blood viscosity, prevents muscle fatigue and cramps, and is a major contributor to skin cooling, which keeps the core body temperature at an optimal level.

Athletes lose two to three liters of water per hour during exercise. To ensure optimal performance, and to maintain overall health, that water must be replenished. Water should not be used by parents or coaches as a reward or goal. It should not be withheld until a certain number of sprints have been finished, or as punishment for poor performance. As parents and coaches, we need to educate our children on the benefits of hydration, as well as about the warning signs of dehydration. Just as it's important for youth athletes to learn baseball drills and skills, it's crucial for them to know how the body works and how to care for it. Water should be readily available during all athletic activity, and water breaks should be programmed into all practice schedules, especially if the environment is high-risk.

How to Hydrate

Coaches, parents, and athletic trainers should encourage their athletes to hydrate prior to activity. This process begins about seventy-two hours in advance of competition, but hydration should be thought of as a good maintenance practice to be included in the daily routine. The FDA recommends drinking six to eight eight-ounce glasses of water per day for a normal, healthy lifestyle. This recommendation is universal and is a good practice to keep the body in peak physical condition.

During activity, athletes should rehydrate with six ounces of fluid every fifteen minutes. Sports drinks are fine, but keep in mind that most sports drinks contain large amounts of sugar that are not necessary to hydration. In a very hot or humid setting, too much sports drink can cause nausea, bloating, and diarrhea. Water is usually sufficient for hydration.

Remember: If You're Thirsty, It's Too Late!

- **Pre-Hydrate:** Begin seventy-two hours in advance of competition
- **Hydrate During Activity:** Six ounces every fifteen minutes
- **Rehydrate:** Drink thirty-two ounces of liquid per one pound of fluid loss

What Is a "High-Risk" Environment?

A high-risk environment is one in which external conditions increase an athlete's chances for heat-related illness by inhibiting the body's ability to cool itself. How does the body cool itself during activity? With sweat! The main function of sweat is to keep the core body temperature down through a process known as evaporative cooling. It may sound complex, but it is actually quite intuitive. When our body temperature rises during activity, it elevates from the core and disperses out through the skin. As sweat evaporates, it provides a cooling mechanism that draws heat away from the body. When this mechanism is functioning normally, as it does in most healthy individuals, it protects us from heat-related illnesses.

Abnormal functioning of the body's evaporative cooling system can cause core body temperature to rise to potentially fatal levels. Some risk factors that can cause the body's evaporative cooling system to malfunction can be controlled, while others cannot. We need to take care of the ones we can control, and properly manage the ones we cannot. As coaches, players, and parents, we need to be aware of the dangers and manage the risk factors that elevate the chances of heat-related illness.

Internal Risk Factors for Heat-Related Illness

Dehydration: This is the first warning sign of potential heat illness. Rule of thumb: if you're thirsty, it's too late! Since our blood is 90 percent water, lower water volume will cause the blood to become thick and viscous, which makes it more difficult for the heart to pump blood to the muscles and organs.

High Body Mass Index, or BMI: Athletes who are overweight or have a higher BMI will have a more difficult time cooling themselves because the excess fat traps heat inside the body. While a BMI chart does not take into account lean muscle mass, they are a quick and easy way to get a general idea of what proper BMI range should be.

Improper Acclimatization: It takes the body anywhere from three to fourteen days to be properly acclimated to a new environment.

It is important for coaches to realize that athletes will not be able to perform as well, and are at a higher risk for heat illness, in the first days of practice, when the body may still be adjusting to climate change.

Heart Disease: Any athlete known to have a heart condition prior to activity must analyze the risks of putting the heart under the increased stresses created by physical activity. This is generally determined by a physician during a pre-participation exam, and overseen by an athletic trainer, coach, or parent.

Hypertension: High blood pressure forces the heart to pump harder and faster. During physical activity, the heart is already under extra stress, and heat and improper hydration can increase that stress.

External Risk Factors for Heat-Related Illness

High Heat Index: The heat index combines air temperature with relative humidity to determine an apparent temperature—that is, how hot does it actually feel?

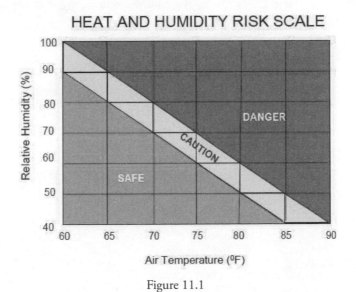

Figure 11.1

Humid Air: When there is excessive moisture in the air, it prohibits evaporation of moisture from the skin, which inhibits the body's evaporative cooling process.

Saturated Clothing: Saturated clothing against the skin also prohibits evaporation of moisture from the skin, which inhibits the body's evaporative cooling process.

Signs and Symptoms of Heat-Related Illness

There are three main types of heat illness: heat cramps, heat exhaustion, and heat syncope (also known as heatstroke), which is fainting as a result of heat-related illness. All are brought about with exertion and lengthened heat exposure, and, generally, with unsafe environmental stressors as contributing factors. Each condition varies in severity, and they usually occur in succession from one to the next.

As mentioned above, physical exertion in a high-risk environment will decrease the body's ability to thermoregulate via evaporative cooling. Even with proper hydration, continuing to physically stress the body in a risky environment is potentially hazardous. This is essentially the mechanism of injury when looking at heat illness, which can be intensified with multiple risk factors. Listed in the below chart are some common signs and symptoms of each heat-related illness, and what to do if they occur.

ILLNESS	SIGNS AND SYMPTOMS	TREATMENT
Heat Cramps	Involuntary muscle contraction	• Remove from play • Stretch muscle for immediate relief • Rehydration
Heat Exhaustion	• Skin redness • Profuse sweating • Nausea • Vomiting	• Medical Emergency • Rehydration • Ice bags around core (under arms, groin, chest, neck)
Heat Syncope	• Complete inability to thermoregulate • Pale/clammy skin • Sweating has ceased • Dizziness • Nausea • Unconsciousness	• Medical Emergency • This individual needs to be rapidly cooled in an ice bath and transported to a trauma center

Heat Cramps

Heat cramps are an early warning sign that heat stress is developing. They most often occur in the lower extremities. Most competitive athletes will try to continue participation, sometimes by rehydrating orally or intravenously, where available. However, it is important to stop activity, rest in a cool place, and rehydrate! Sports beverages help replenish electrolytes lost through sweat. If cramping does not improve within an hour, seek medical attention, as they can rapidly accelerate into a life-threatening problem. Furthermore, continuing to play with a cramped muscle increases the risk of a muscle strain or tear.

Heat Exhaustion

At this stage, the athlete will experience heavy sweating, skin redness, and, possibly, even nausea or vomiting. There can also be symptoms that mimic those of a concussion: headache, blurred vision, dizziness, and, possibly, fainting. It's important to understand that heat exhaustion is life threatening! Call 911 immediately. Rapid cooling is crucial. Ice baths are recommended if available and, at the very least, saturated clothing should be removed to help bring the core body temperature back to a safe level.

Heat Syncope or Heatstroke

At this point, the body is completely unable to thermoregulate, or control its own temperature. The body is no longer producing sweat, the skin is red hot, and the athlete is often in an altered mental state. Fainting is a possibility. Body temperature can be upwards of 104 degrees within ten minutes of identifying heat illness and, if left untreated, can result in permanent damage to the brain or other vital organs and, possibly, even death. Heatstroke kills close to four thousand Americans per year, so once symptoms are identified, it is important to call 911 and take immediate action to cool the body. This is best achieved with an ice bath, or with ice packs or cold sponges under the armpits and knees and at the groin. Do not give any liquids or solids by mouth.

NUTRITION

Baseball nutrition must be approached with common sense and an understanding of what it means to properly fuel for competition. I always get a kick out of athletes who can't connect what they're eating during the day with their performance on the field.

Youth and teenage athletes must develop good eating habits that will last them a lifetime. This is the best time to introduce a healthy lifestyle so they make the connection between input and output. What we put into our bodies is directly linked to what we get out of our bodies. A bag of chips won't get you through a doubleheader in the hot afternoon sun. Good nutrition not only benefits the baseball athlete or the youth athlete; healthy eating habits are important for people of every age and form the foundation for healthy living.

Macronutrients

There are three basic macronutrients that comprise the basis of our diet: carbohydrates, proteins, and fats. Each macronutrient is essential in its own right and is a necessary component for a healthy, well-rounded diet. Every meal should include items from each category, whether a person is trying to maintain, lose, or gain weight. Depending on an athlete's nutritional goals, meals may be added or subtracted throughout the day.

A basic guideline is to eat meals consisting of 65 percent carbohydrate, 20 percent protein and 15 percent fat. Of course, estimations can be made, but the only true way to accomplish this is to weigh our food.

Baseball players should use a checklist to aid in getting these percentages into their meals and into their body. A healthy-eating checklist can include the following:

- Eat breakfast seven days a week
- Eat three to four balanced meals at the same time each day
- Have a nutritious mid-morning snack
- Eat two to three pieces of fresh fruit per day
- Eat four to five servings of fresh vegetables each day (not out of a can!)
- Eat breads or cereals high in fiber
- Eat lean, low-fat proteins (chicken, tuna, steak) at each meal
- Maintain body weight (goal dependent)
- Have a nutritious snack an hour before a workout
- Have a nutritious snack thirty to forty-five minutes post-workout
- Eat a well-balanced meal two to three hours before competition
- Hydrate appropriately throughout the day
- Take a daily multivitamin

It is very important that athletes realize that proper, consistent nutrition will help them perform at a high level. It will also help the body heal more quickly, which allows the athlete to consistently participate and stay fit throughout the season. Proper nutrition and hydration can also decrease the risk of muscular injuries, which is what this book is about.

Carbohydrates

Carbohydrates are the first energy source expended by the body during activity. They are easily mobilized and directly available in the bloodstream. Our skeletal muscle needs this quick energy source readily available throughout activity. As we see from marathon runners and their prerace pasta parties, carbohydrates are necessary to sustain peak performance.

However, if you are not training and burning off carbohydrates as energy, they will eventually be stored as fat. Understand that these guidelines are for athletes training for baseball-specific activity, with competitions equally as long. Non-baseball player guidelines will be slightly different, but only in the amount of intake.

There are three types of carbohydrates that can be derived from our food choices: slow-, moderate-, and fast-absorbing carbohydrates. Each has its place, and must be included in a well-balanced diet.

Fast-Absorbing Carbohydrates

Fast-absorbing carbs can be used for quick energy almost immediately after consumption. This includes: waffles, pancakes, potatoes, bagels, sport drinks, corn chips, and some fruit, such as watermelon, cantaloupe, and pineapple. These are all high in sugar, and not always the best choice of carbohydrate. The best time to eat these is prior to athletic activity, and immediately post-exercise to replenish lost carbohydrate stores. But, beware, because the body burns these carbohydrates so quickly, a "crash" can result if the body is not properly fueled with other foods at regular intervals throughout the day.

Moderate-Absorbing Carbohydrates

These carbs are the in-between choices that absorb just a little more slowly than those in the fast-absorbing category. Examples include: whole-grain breads, high-fiber cereal, brown rice, pasta, oatmeal, sweet potatoes, fruit juice, bananas, grapes, and raisins.

Slow-Absorbing Carbohydrates

Slow-absorbing carbs are good for long-term maintenance of carbohydrate levels. They are good to include pre-activity to increase energy stores for the long term so they are readily available when they're needed.

Examples include: apples, cherries, peaches, plums, pears, chickpeas, milk, yogurt, eggplant, broccoli, and brussels sprouts.

Protein

Protein is important for the restoration of muscle fibers following the breakdown that occurs with exercise. Protein choice is based on how the body breaks it down. First-choice protein sources include: lean meats, such as fat-trimmed beef or pork, chicken, white tuna in water, and non-fried seafood. Second choice sources come from: dairy, nuts and seeds, milk, soy milk, yogurt, beans, peas, lentils, soy foods, and peanut butter.

Fat

Fat is the secondary source of energy, and is often used during long bouts of exercise or activity. It is an essential part of the body's composition and must be included in the athlete's diet. Many diet and nutritional books advocate avoiding fats, but realize: the body needs fats to protect the organs and maximize athletic composition. Of course, there are good fats and bad fats. Saturated fat is the bad fat the body does not need, most often found in fried foods, fast foods, and in animal fats such as cheese, cream, and butter. Polyunsaturated fat should be limited, and is found in vegetable oils and processed margarine. The best fat is monounsaturated fat, found in: whole foods such as olives, extra-virgin olive oil, avocados, fish, clams, oysters, scallops, nuts, and natural peanut butter.

Caloric Intake

The essential thing to understand about caloric intake is the simple concept of input versus output. Calories measure the energy value of a food product. An athlete's caloric intake for the day is dictated by how much energy will be expended that day. A high-activity day requires higher consumption. Conversely, a low-activity day will not have as much caloric demand and consumption should be lower.

If an athlete is programming for weight loss or gain, caloric intake may need to be further adjusted. Baseline caloric intake can be calculated by multiplying body weight in pounds times fifteen. For example, a

150-pound athlete must consume 2,250 calories per day to maintain current body weight. Work from this baseline to accommodate for higher- and lower-activity days, and adjust the total caloric intake based on goals of weight gain or loss.

SUPPLEMENT AND STEROID ABUSE IN THE BASEBALL PLAYER

Everything an athlete might gain from supplementation can be achieved through proper nutrition. However, a busy, active lifestyle can make it difficult to always eat a proper meal. Subsequently, athletes may have a hard time obtaining all the proper daily nutrients from food choices alone and may look to supplementation to bridge this gap. It is always wise to consult a physician who knows your medical background and can make an educated recommendation about supplementation before deciding on a product to use. Keep in mind that the FDA does not regulate the dietary supplement industry, which means it is impossible to truly know what you are putting into your body. This is especially important if competing in the NCAA and throughout the professional sport leagues, as there may be a banned substance in the manufacturer's "proprietary blend" that can cause drug test failure. Even more importantly, if you don't know what you're putting into your body, you may be putting yourself at a major health risk.

Human beings should not add anything into their diets if they don't know exactly what it is, especially if a physician or nutritionist does not guide the decision. Too many times, decisions are made by looking in the mirror, and not by getting the appropriate urinalysis to see if the body is indeed lacking any nutrients. It's my opinion that you should not put any man-made supplements into your body unless approved after testing. Research shows that 65–75 percent of added vitamins and minerals cannot be properly absorbed and literally end up in the toilet bowl. Basically, you're flushing your money down the toilet.

Many athletes want to use some sort of protein or creatine supplement to add muscle mass and aid in muscle recovery. These products can safely be used for exactly those reasons, but it is important for athletes to understand that more is not always better, especially because supplement abuse can sometimes lead to steroid abuse.

Harmful Effects of Supplementation and Steroid Abuse

Think of the body as a storage room with shelves. Look at the different nutrients on each labeled shelf. The body, through foods and a multivitamin, will fill each shelf accordingly. Once the shelves are full, the body cannot absorb any more and will have to work harder to flush out the excess. Oversupplementation can overstress the digestive system, liver, stomach, and pancreas, and can potentially result in damage to the system.

A more immediate threat comes from products acting as "accelerants." These products claim to help the body get lean or more "cut." Common sense says if you're taking something to speed up metabolism, and your heart rate along with it, your heart will eventually get tired and fail. Why would anyone, especially athletes, want to speed up their heart prior to exercise? This is a major risk for any athlete and should never be a part of anyone's diet.

Unfortunately, some baseball athletes will skip over the supplement stage and jump directly into steroid use. It is important to understand that steroids are drugs. They are man-made substances related to the male sex hormone testosterone. Medically, some are used for various pathologies and can be used for good, but, when abused by athletes, steroids always cause more harm than good.

People use the big words "anabolic," or "muscle-building," and "androgenic," which refers to masculine characteristics, when describing steroids. Athletes are always looking for an edge, and steroids will give you that edge. You will get bigger, faster and stronger, but not without harmful, unavoidable side effects.

Side Effects of Steroids in Males
- Shrinking testicles
- Infertility
- Baldness
- Increased breast size
- Increased risk of cancer

Side Effects of Steroids in Females
- Changes to the menstrual cycle
- Deepened voice

- Male characteristics such as facial hair or male-pattern baldness
- Long-term effects from depleted estrogen
- Infertility
- Increased risk of cancer

Other harmful effects of steroids in children and young athletes are accelerated puberty, premature growth and shortened growth plates, liver tumors, fluid retention, increase in LDL or bad cholesterol, decrease in HDL or good cholesterol, kidney tumors, severe acne, and tremors. If steroids are injected, HIV and AIDS are also risks. Steroids can also have psychological effects, such as aggression, mood swings, and invincibility traits.

I understand that baseball athletes face pressure from a variety of sources. Parents, coaches, peers, and teammates expect the athlete to perform. The athlete wants to get a scholarship or financial aid or "go pro," and he or she may view supplements and steroids as a shortcut to success. But steroids are drugs, and they are illegal, and using them at any level is cheating. If an athlete feels he or she needs an additional edge, there are nutrition professionals available for consultation. They're all able to help athletes achieve their nutritional goals and maximize their athletic potential. But, remember, nothing can replace hard work!

CHAPTER 12
by John Gallucci, Jr.

BIOMECHANICS AND CORE DEVELOPMENT FOR THE BASEBALL PLAYER

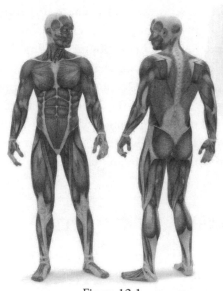

Figure 12.1

A well-trained and well-developed core is essential for optimal performance and injury prevention. The body's core region is often referred to as the torso or trunk, which implies that it involves more than just the abdominal muscles. The major muscles involved in core stability include the pelvic floor muscles, transverse abdominis, multifidus, internal and external obliques, rectus abdominis, erector spinae, and the diaphragm. The minor muscles include the latissimus dorsi, gluteus maximus, gluteus medius, and the trapezius. Core exercises train the muscles in your pelvis, lower back, hips, and abdomen to work in harmony. This leads to better balance and stability, whether on the playing field or in daily activities. All sports, and many other physical activities, depend on stable and strong core muscles.

To visualize the importance of the core, envision your core muscles as the central link in a chain that connects your upper and lower body. Whether you're swinging a bat or running the bases, the respective motions either originate in your core, or move through it.

Regardless of where the force originates, it travels upward and downward to adjoining links of the chain. This chain reaction relies on all links in the chain to handle the load of the forces. Weak or inflexible core muscles can impair the process of transferring force through the chain. Therefore, underdeveloped core muscles can affect how well your arms and legs function. Insufficient core muscles do not allow the forces that act on the body to properly transfer down or up the chain. That, in turn, drains power from many of the moves you make. Properly building up their core allows individuals to generate and transfer more power. Additionally, strong core muscles enhance balance and stability, which can help prevent falls and injuries during sports or other activities.

Weak, tight, or unbalanced core muscles can undermine your efforts to get stronger or faster. And while it's important to build a strong core, it would also be a mistake to focus all your efforts on developing rippling abs. Overtraining abdominal muscles while ignoring muscles of the back and hips can increase injury and limit athletic ability. Developing a strong core is crucial to becoming the best athlete you can be. The important thing to remember when developing the core is that the abdominal muscles are not the only muscle group within the core. The back, hips, and pelvis must also be addressed when developing a core-strengthening program.

THE CORE AND THE BASEBALL ATHLETE

The core, as it relates to baseball, plays a large role in performance. The most obvious functions of the core muscles are their role in rotating the body for swinging the bat or throwing the ball. There is another function, however: the transfer energy, which translates to transfer of power. The legs generate the initial speed and power of the movements most associated with baseball, but the core helps transfer that power through the torso and into the arms and hands of the athlete. It is this mechanism that dramatically increases bat speed for hitters, as arm speed and velocity is generated for pitchers. In this chapter, we will focus on the biomechanics of baseball movements and how they stem from a strong, stable core.

THE BIOMECHANICS OF THE THROW OR PITCH

The overhand pitching motion includes a sequence of body movements that originate when the pitcher lifts the lead foot, progresses to a linked motion in the hips and trunk, and ultimately results in an explosive motion of the upper extremity to propel the ball toward home plate. The effective synchronized use of selective muscle groups maximizes the efficiency of the kinetic chain. The lower extremity and trunk generate and transfer energy to the upper extremity. Coordinated lower extremity muscles (quadriceps, hamstrings, and hip internal and external rotators) provide a stable base for the trunk (core musculature) to rotate and flex. Typically, the time between foot strike and ball release is under 0.2 seconds.

A pitcher's velocity, consistency, and durability derive from a development of many kinematic factors, as well as the efficient transfer of energy to the sequence of segmented body motions. Optimizing these parameters relies on a stable and strong core. There cannot be an efficient and consistent transfer of energy from proximal to distal components without a cohesive kinematic effort through the trunk. Understanding the variables that optimize function may prevent injury by reducing the leak of energy through the kinetic chain, which results in dysfunction in related movements. A breakdown of the kinetic chain will reduce its efficiency, making top velocity, control, and durability more difficult to achieve.

THE SIX PHASES OF A PITCH

The pitching motion consists of six phases. The phases are the wind-up, early cocking/stride, late cocking, acceleration, deceleration, and the follow-through. These phases are intricately connected. Successfully connecting all phases of the throwing motion efficiently generates and transfers energy from the body into the arm, the hand, and the ball. The wind-up and stride position rely on the lower extremity and trunk for optimal performance of the kinetic chain. The legs and trunk serve as the main force generators of the kinetic chain. The complex interaction of the lower extremities and core musculature in the kinetic chain reduces the kinetic contributions of the shoulder joint. When this occurs properly, the pitching motion should not be considered purely an upper extremity action, but, rather, an integrated motion of the entire body that ultimately allows for rapid motion of the upper extremity. Athletes can improve velocity by optimizing the kinetic chain, which also reduces the shoulder's kinetic contributions necessary to produce that velocity. Reduced kinetic stresses on the shoulder may prevent injury, leading to greater durability and health of the throwing shoulder.

The Wind-up Phase

The wind-up phase positions the body to generate the forces and power required to achieve top velocity. The wind-up begins with the initial movement of the opposite (to the throwing arm) lower extremity, and it culminates with elevation of the lead leg to its highest point and the throwing hand separating from the glove. The pitcher keeps the center of gravity over the back leg to generate maximum momentum once forward motion is initiated. Weakness in the core leads to the pitcher's body and momentum falling forward prematurely. As a result, the kinetic chain will be disrupted and greater shoulder force is required to propel the ball at top velocity. During the wind-up, pitchers must hold their center of gravity toward the back (over their stance leg) for as long as possible to allow maximum generation and transfer of momentum and force to the upper extremity and ball.

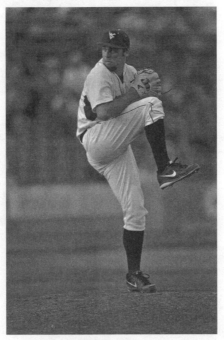

Figure 12.2

The Early Cocking/Stride Phase

The early cocking/stride phase begins once the lead leg reaches its maximum height and the ball exits the glove. This phase ends when the lead foot contacts the pitching mound. The stride increases the distance over which linear and angular trunk motions occur, allowing increased energy production to transfer through the core to the upper extremity. The knee and hip of the stance leg extend to begin pelvic rotation and forward tilt, followed by upper torso rotation. The abdominal obliques eccentrically contract to prevent excess lumbar hyperextension during upper torso rotation and flexion. This is one of the stabilizing roles of the core to prevent energy leaks in the kinetic chain. The gluteus maximus of the stance leg fires to maintain slight extension and provide pelvis and trunk stabilization during coiling. The lead foot should land in line with the stance foot, pointing toward home plate.

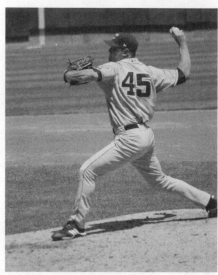

Figure 12.3

The Late Cocking Phase

The late cocking phase occurs between lead foot contact and the point of maximal external rotation of the throwing shoulder. The late cocking phase can be observed as the scapula is brought into a position of retraction, the elbow flexes, and the humerus undergoes abduction and external rotation. It is also at this point that the pelvis reaches its maximum rotation and the upper torso continues to rotate and tilt forward and laterally. In this phase, the lead knee begins to extend, forming a solid base for trunk flexion. As the torso rotates, the throwing arm is pulled into horizontal adduction. The final stage of the cocking phase is where the maximum valgus torque is experienced at the elbow. As the pitcher finishes the late cocking phase, the arm is positioned at 95 degrees of elbow flexion, 165 to 175 degrees of external rotation, 90 to 95 degrees of abduction, and 10 to 20 degrees horizontal adduction. In this phase, most of the mechanical movements occur in the upper extremity, but the core and trunk must maintain their role of stabilizing the pitcher through the entire phase. Breakdowns in the core in earlier phases can lead to dysfunction in the late cocking phase— the phase where the shoulder and elbow experience the greatest amount of force.

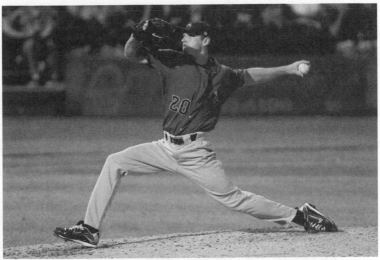

Figure 12.4

The Acceleration Phase

The acceleration phase is defined as the time between maximum external rotation of the shoulder and ball release. The trunk continues to rotate and tilt, initiating the transfer of potential energy through the upper extremity. The scapula protracts to maintain a stable base as the humerus is moved into horizontal adduction and rapid internal rotation. This motion delivers the arm from as much as 175 degrees of external rotation to 100 degrees of internal rotation (at ball release) in a very short amount of time—under half a second. The non-dominant rectus abdominus, abdominal obliques, and lumbar paraspinal muscles must activate during acceleration to emphasize pelvic and trunk rotation and tilt. Concentric rectus femoris contraction contributes to lead leg hip flexion and knee extension, providing a stable front side to facilitate increased angular momentum of the trunk. Increased forward trunk tilt allows the pitching arm to accelerate over a greater distance, which allows more force to be transferred to the ball.

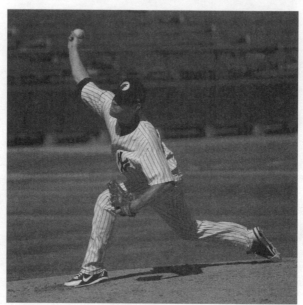

Figure 12.5

The Deceleration Phase

The deceleration phase occurs between ball release and maximum humeral internal rotation and elbow extension. Deceleration is the phase that is the most violent of the throwing cycle. This creates the greatest potential for injury due to the amount of joint loading during throwing. Essentially, this phase releases all the energy generated during the previous phases. The posterior shoulder musculature is essential in dissipating the forces that are generated. The trapezius, rhomboids, and serratus anterior must activate to stabilize the scapula during deceleration. Once the ball is released, core activation prevents the body from over-rotating and allows for proper deceleration. Since there is so much force placed on the upper extremity during deceleration, the functions of the core are essential for a safe retransfer of energy. A weak core could result in lagging recovery, which could cause injury in various kinematic links in the chain. If the core is unable to stabilize the trunk through deceleration, it could result in a breakdown in the back, shoulder, or elbow due to the nature of the force generated.

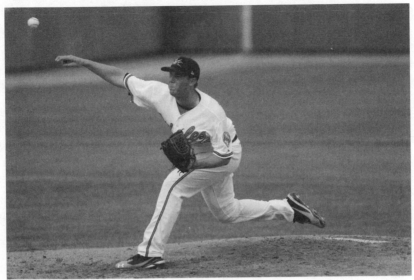

Figure 12.6

The Follow-through Phase of Pitching

The follow-through is an extension of the deceleration phase where the body continues to move forward with the arm until motion is finished. The body relaxes during the follow-through and eases overall loading on

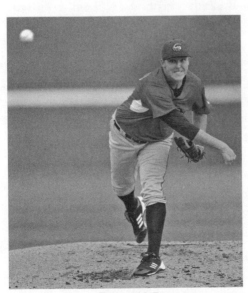

Figure 12.7

the joints. The shoulder and arm experience the greatest change in overall energy. The lower extremity and core are still responsible for stabilizing the body. After the massive energy release, the muscles of the trunk and lower extremity continue to contract to provide a base of support. Once the pitch is complete, the job is not done. The follow-through phase ends with the pitcher standing in a fielding position, ready to react.

THE BIOMECHANICS OF BATTING

The hitting motion consists of five phases. Each phase is built on the previous phase, creating a cohesive sequence of movements. These movements, much like the pitching motion, occur through a series of movements in the kinetic chain. The effective synchronized use of selective muscle groups maximizes the efficiency of the kinetic chain. The lower extremity and trunk generate and transfer energy to the upper extremity. Coordination of the lower extremity muscles provides a stable base for the trunk and core to allow for proper trunk flexion and rotation. Hitting properly stems from a development of many kinetic factors, as well as the efficient transfer of energy to the sequence of segmented body motions. Optimizing these parameters relies on a stable and strong core. There cannot be an efficient and consistent transfer of energy from proximal to distal components without a cohesive kinetic effort through the trunk. The five phases of hitting are the stance, the loading phase, the timing mechanism, the launching phase, and the follow-through. (All explanations are for a right-handed batter.)

The Stance

The stance requires placement of the feet slightly wider than shoulder width. The weight is balanced and evenly distributed through both feet. Unlike the pitching phases, the stance does not require specific hand placement or shoulder angle. In this phase, the key is to be comfortable and balanced. The balanced stance relies on the musculature of the lower extremity to stabilize the batter. The knees should be slightly bent and locked solidly into position. The hips should be squarely underneath, and directly in line with, the shoulders. The line between each shoulder and hip should be parallel. The lower back should not be arched, and the butt should not be sticking out. The positioning of the hips and the neutrality of the spine are reliant on a strong and stable core. Control of the trunk is essential throughout the swing, and the ability to swing properly is dependent on the core control established in the stance.

The Loading Phase

The loading phase begins with the backward movement of the shoulders and arms. The left arm undergoes adduction through activation of the pectoralis major, latissimus dorsi, and the teres major. While this occurs, it conversely causes the posterior (closer to catcher) shoulder (posterior deltoid, rhomboid, and trapezius) to load. The right arm abducts or moves away from the body through activation of the supraspinatus and the middle deltoid. This loads the latissimus dorsi, teres major, pectoralis major, and serratus anterior with potential energy. The next area of focus in the loading phase is the backward rotation of the spine. This occurs with the activation of the external abdominal oblique, rotatores spinea, and the multifidus muscles. The loading phase also includes the beginning of the timing step. As soon as the backward movement of the shoulder and arms occurs, so does the beginning of the timing step. This forces the back leg in the stance to carry the weight of the batter. This allows the hip extensors, hamstring, and calf muscles on the rear leg to load. The rotation of the shoulders and spine combined with the weight transfer to the back foot allows the hips to cock. This cocking motion stretches the hip external rotators (gluteus maximus, gluteus medius, piriformis, obturator externus, and quadratus femoris), allowing them to load. The cocking of the hips stores the elastic energy required to launch into an effective swing. The primary loading occurs in the hips and trunk, which allows for a coiling effect in the body. The core is responsible for storing this potential energy and is the primary loading factor in the swing.

The Timing Mechanism/Transition Phase

The timing mechanism is defined as one's ability to initiate the transition from the loading phase into the launching phase, so that should you decide to swing, you will have enough time to get the bat around to make good contact with the ball. In the loading phase, the arms and shoulders bring the bat back into position. However, this position is not the farthest point the bat will go back. During the timing mechanism, or "transition phase," the shoulders, arms, and wrists are in the loading phase and the hips and legs begin the explosive forward rotation that defines the launching phase. As the hips rotate forward, the timing step is also beginning its return to the ground. It is at this point, as the hips begin to rotate, that the shoulders and arms actually rotate back even farther, generating more potential energy in the bat. The timing mechanism is a very short phase and is identifiable by the movement of the hips and final backward movement of the bat.

The Launching Phase

The launching phase begins when the timing step returns to the ground, which opens up the hips. Since a majority of one's batting power comes from hip rotation, the repositioning of the timing step, where the toes are now pointing outward or toward first base, is necessary since this starts the opening of both hips toward the pitcher, which is the direction the batter will end up facing at contact. The external rotation of the hips is caused by activation of the hip's internal rotators (gluteus medius and tensor fascia lata). This is where the generation of power begins. The potential energy generated while loading is now being unleashed in the form of hip and spinal rotation. Once the hips begin their rotation, the back leg begins its push up to assist further in rotational power. The right foot plantar flexes into the ground, which generates a reciprocal force through the lower extremity and travels through the kinetic chain. The knee and hips also extend to allow the energy to travel directly into the trunk as it rotates. All the rotational forces are transferred through the trunk and are facilitated by the core musculature. There can be no rotation of the body without a strong and stable core. The energy transfer from the back leg into the core allows the hips to rotate even faster than allowed by the potential energy generated during loading. As the energy transfer progresses through the kinetic chain, the next links are the spine, chest, and shoulders. The external oblique, multifidus, and rotatores spinea muscles on the left side of the body activate to allow the upper extremity to rotate toward the pitcher. As the spine and shoulders are forced into the launching phase, the next and final movements occur in the arms and, ultimately, the bat. The bat head is actually the last link in the chain where all the centrifugal force is directed and stored. The loading phase culminates at ball strike.

The Follow-through Phase in Batting

The follow-through is the time after contact with the ball. It continues the rotation in the hips and spine, as well as pushing and pulling the arms. The follow-through involves a lot of deceleration of the body's movements. The momentum of the swing carries the batter into a position of internal rotation of the hips. It is, again, the core musculature that must contract to stabilize these movements. The antagonistic contractions of the hips and core rotators slow the body and shoulders of the batter. This allows the batter to change position from hitting to running to first base. The batter cannot effectively follow through without a stable core to slow the rotational forces in an efficient way. The swing is completed during the follow-through as the batter begins the run to first base.

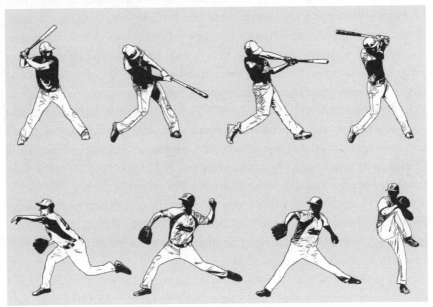

Figure 12.8

CHAPTER 13
by John Gallucci, Jr.

STRENGTH AND CONDITIONING

When athletes define their fitness goals, they must take into account what attributes are desirable for their chosen sport. Baseball athletes will not train the same way as power lifters, who will not train the same way as swimmers. So, what abilities or traits give the ideal baseball player success on the field? Power. Speed. Quickness. Agility. Flexibility. Strength. Stamina. Balance.

Baseball athletes must include a good strength and conditioning program to improve these attributes across the board. The program should target the athlete's weaknesses in order to improve them.

If time is invested in strength and conditioning on a daily basis, many injuries can be prevented, especially over the course of a long season when the body needs to be in peak condition. Our goal as fitness professionals is to improve the athlete's foundational fitness attributes away from the field through a logical strength and conditioning program.

Of course, baseball players also have incredible, sport-specific skills, such as fast-acting hand-eye coordination. No amount of time in the gym will prepare an athlete for what happens on the field. To get better at baseball, we need to get out and play it!

Though fitness is always a goal for athletes, it is equally important for the athlete to be competing on a regular basis. Competition is the force that drives us to better ourselves and hone our skills over the course of time.

The objective of this chapter is to provide athletes with a framework for a good strength and conditioning program so they may design and implement their own. It is important to organize the program in a logical progression to lay the foundation for success in baseball. The reason for such a generalized approach is that there is no single program that can give you the speed, strength, and ability to guarantee success in baseball.

However, it is important to be knowledgeable in your approach to strength and conditioning, and to understand planning and goal setting as it relates to a strength and conditioning program.

ENERGY SYSTEMS

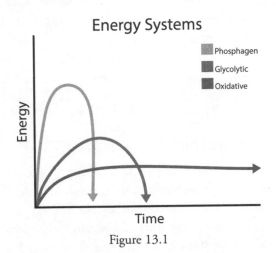

Figure 13.1

What fuels an athlete? There are three energy systems, or bioenergetics, that overlap and work together on a cellular level to physiologically produce energy and effectively fuel our bodies during activity. Two of the systems, the phosphagen and glycolytic systems, are anaerobic, which run in the absence of oxygen. The third system, the aerobic system, operates in the presence of oxygen. All these run on different time frames, offering varying intensity levels lasting from several seconds to hours.

Anaerobic Systems

Currently available energy molecules present in our skeletal muscle, known as ATP, or adenosine triphosphate, fuel anaerobic systems. ATP is used during exercise, takes time to replenish, and does so only in the presence of oxygen. In the short term, there is a limited supply. Thus, when the body is operating anaerobically, rapid exhaustion results from the limited supply of energy molecules.

The Phosphagen System

During short-term, intense bursts of exercise—e.g., stealing a base—the muscles need to produce a lot of power, which creates huge demand for ATP, making the phosphagen system the quickest synthesizer of ATP. Because this system runs in the absence of oxygen, and the body relies on oxygen for nearly everything it does, and because the body has a limited supply of ATP molecules, we cannot last very long within this system. Exercise fueled by the phosphagen system only lasts about ten seconds before exhaustion. This is high-intensity exercise and requires maximal effort. Sample exercises include single rep max-effort power lifts and meter sprints.

The Glycolytic System

This system is in the mid-range and lies between the phosphagen and aerobic systems. It is the second-fastest synthesizer of ATP. During this phase, blood glucose is broken down and usable ATP is produced. Exercise fueled by this system lasts in the thirty-second to two-minute range before exhaustion. Sample exercises include 100-meter sprints with time allowed for recovery or running around the bases.

The Aerobic System

The aerobic system is the most complex of the three energy systems. It is run in the presence of oxygen. "Aerobic" means "requiring air." While this system produces the most ATP, it also synthesizes it slowly. This means the aerobic system can't fuel exercise that requires the fast production of ATP, but, at a steadier pace, its capacity is virtually inexhaustible. This is the body's primary energy system; it is constantly churning and replenishes the other two systems. Aerobic exercises are of long duration and low intensity. Examples include long-distance running, biking, or swimming.

It is important to remember that these energy systems are not independent of one another. They all work and run simultaneously during activity. However, depending on the specific demands placed on an athlete, one energy system may be taxed more than the others over the course of a practice, game, or training session. It is therefore important to stress each system on a weekly, and even daily, basis in training to be ready for every athletic situation. Since the aerobic system is always churning, it is possible to increase aerobic capacity in an anaerobic training environment. For example, both a five-mile run and multiple 100-meter sprints will increase aerobic capacity.

THE PHYSICAL DEMANDS OF BASEBALL

High school baseball games typically run for about two to two and a half hours. Even though the game may be long, and different positions require different skills, baseball athletes generally rely on the short-term, quick bursts of energy provided by their anaerobic systems more than their aerobic system. Of course, due to the length of the game, over the course of game-play, the athlete will also dip into the anaerobic system energy stores.

Fitness must be improved in all systems for athletes to make overall gains. Training regimens must be varied to incorporate the different phases and expected demands of baseball. Through constant variation, athletes can prepare their bodies for any unknown challenge thrown their way.

Baseball athletes must be fit for baseball. That fitness includes overall health. The fittest athlete is not only the one who is able to compete at the highest level, but also the one who is able to compete in the most competitions over the course of a long season. Losing time to injury is often unavoidable, but athletes can limit their time away from the diamond by taking care of their bodies as much as possible.

TARGET TRAINING ZONES

Athletes should target between 60 percent and 85 percent of their maximum heart rate through the course of their training. Various studies show us that athletes training in this range, from thirty to forty-five minutes per day, are truly working at an aerobic threshold, which will improve their endurance, lung capacity, and general fitness. As stated earlier, it is equally beneficial to train for shorter durations at higher intensities, stressing the various energy pathways in preparation for sport.

A simple formula can be used to determine an athlete's maximum heart rate. By subtracting the athlete's age from 220, we get an estimated maximum heart rate. For example, a fifteen-year-old athlete will have an estimated maximum heart rate of 205 beats per minute (bpm). From this number, we can calculate our training percentages; i.e., 60 percent is 0.60 x 205, or 123 bpm.

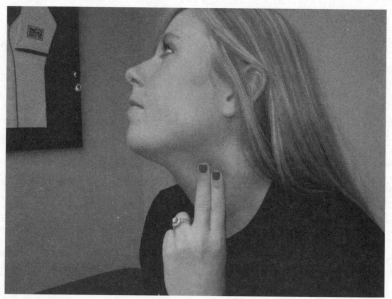

Figure 13.2

Athletes can also take their pulse to check their heart rate during activity, either on the inside of the wrist or at the carotid artery at the side of the neck. Count the number of beats in fifteen seconds and multiply by four. If that's too difficult, just count out the entire minute!

Outside of this guideline, everyone should train within their means with respect to their age to prevent risk of injury.

As athletes train and become more physically fit, they will ultimately see their resting heart rates improve—by decreasing. As determined by the American Heart Association, the resting heart rate of the average individual should be between 60 and 80 bpm. However, elite athletes can fall as low as 35 to 50 bpm.

Anaerobic Training

Hard-core, high-level athletic training usually falls somewhere between 80 percent and 90 percent of an athlete's maximum heart rate. This is the anaerobic training zone. This activity is done in short bursts: from just seconds all the way up to about two minutes. This training is used to promote strength. It is important to train in this zone to help build muscle mass and improve speed and explosiveness.

During or immediately following an anaerobic activity, athletes sometimes describe a burning sensation in the muscle, weakness or "heavy" extremities, and cramping. This uncomfortable, but most certainly temporary, feeling is the buildup of lactic acid, or lactate, which can be converted into energy in the absence of oxygen. Lactic acid builds up faster than it can be "burned off," leading to the above-described symptoms.

Sample exercises include short sprints, hills, and explosive jumps that build the overall body strength crucial to an athlete in the last inning of a game when muscles are thoroughly fatigued.

Aerobic Training

Even though baseball athletes aren't running six to seven miles per game as soccer players are, it is still important to train the aerobic system. Aerobic training should be done at around 60 to 75 percent of maximum heart rate. As stated earlier, the aerobic system is constantly running to produce energy and replenish lost energy stores within our muscles. Improving the body's ability to generate and regenerate lost energy stores will improve the body's capacity to reduce lactic acid buildup in the muscles, and will subsequently increase strength and conditioning.

It is my recommendation that athletes should be in the gym or weight room two to three times per week in season and three to four times per week out of season. In-season training is necessary to maintain strength levels throughout the course of a rigorous season, without overtaxing the body. Offseason training should be programmed to improve overall strength and conditioning levels across all competencies. This is when the biggest gains are made.

Make sure off days are scheduled into every strength and conditioning program. The body benefits just as much from rest as it does from work.

My recommendation is to do a full-body strength routine with three sets of ten reps (3 x 10). As the baseball athlete progresses into more formalized programs, strength and conditioning becomes a truly integral part of the training. Licensed strength coaches will teach different levels of rest, periodization, and pyramid systems, as well as other techniques and programs. For the purposes of the young athlete, the larger muscle groups should be broken down: quads, hamstrings, calves, chest, upper back, shoulders, and arms. Some recommended exercises are squats, calf raises, dumbbell rows and raises, push-ups, and bicep curls.

Remember: always have a partner or spotter, even when training at home in the basement. Be sure to get full range of motion in the entire joint for maximum benefit. Range of motion is the distance a lever can move while attached to a fixed point. Imagine your bones as levers and the joints as fixed points, and make sure you exercise them from full flexion to full extension.

Core Training

The core is a very important part of any athlete. But what, exactly, is it? It's basically the torso: the body minus the arms and legs. The core includes all the muscles of the abdomen, the lower back, and the upper hip. These muscles are necessary for continuous spinal stabilization and rotational stability. When the core is strong and stable, many injuries can be prevented. Exercises to improve core strength are not limited to standard flexion or crunch abdominal exercises, but they must also incorporate an extension component. Examples include the superman, done on all fours while raising the arms and legs off the ground. This is a great way to incorporate the back side of the body and maintain balance in the front and back, as well as on both sides.

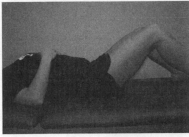

Figure 13.3

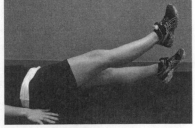

Figure 13.4

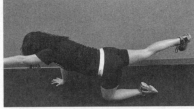

Figure 13.5

Flexibility

Flexibility is a simple and extremely necessary component of every strength and conditioning program. Training causes fatigue in the muscles, which can cause them to tighten. Spasms in tight muscles can cause pain. Too much training can result in overuse injuries. Running athletes are most commonly sore with tight hamstrings and external rotators such as the piriformis and gluteals, and throwing athletes are typically sore in the internal rotators (subscapularis and pectoralis major) and external rotators (infraspinatus and teres minor) of the shoulder. Soreness from training can make everyday activities difficult to perform, but, with adequate flexibility, the activities of daily living are easy.

Flexibility is also a key part of most rehabilitation protocols and is always essential to the prevention of athletic injury.

There are two primary ways athletes can improve their flexibility through standard techniques. In static stretching, muscles are elongated into a stretch that is typically held for a period of thirty seconds. The stretch is usually repeated three times. Though this technique has value and should be included in strength and conditioning programs, dynamic stretching has more benefits than static stretching. Dynamic stretching is a technique that uses a rapid elongation of the muscle followed by a rapid shortening. Examples of dynamic stretches are high-knees, squat jumps, and side-shuffles. This is proven to increase blood flow deep within the muscles, increasing the body temperature and the flexibility of the skeletal muscle.

A good warm-up or cooldown should include both static and dynamic stretching that targets the specific muscles used repeatedly in baseball. Baseball athletes must engage in all sorts of dynamic motion: forward running, backward running, side shuffling, jumping, throwing, and rotating. All these different mechanical motions require different demands at each limb, directed through the torso. It is important to keep these various and specific actions in mind when designing a stretching protocol and strength and conditioning program, as well as when rehabilitating an injury.

I recommend that every athlete do some flexibility work every day. Pre-activity stretches should be done after a ten- to fifteen-minute warm-up during which the athlete has broken a sweat. Post-activity, stretches should be held for twenty to thirty seconds and should address all muscles used during activity, including the quadriceps, hamstrings, piriformis, calves, hip flexors, abdominals, lower back, groin and adductors, IT band, shoulders, neck, and upper back.

BROAD-BASED CONDITIONING PROGRAM

(Perform circuit three days a week with a one-minute break between each rotation.)

- **Warm-up**: Jumping Jacks, High Knees, Butt Kicks, Lateral Hops @ one minute each
- **Cardio Component**: Run two miles three to five times per week

Body Part(s)	Exercise	Sets	Reps
Core	Plank	3	30 sec.
	Side Planks (Bilateral)	3	15 sec.
	Bicycle Crunches	3	30 sec.
Core, Lower Back	Bird Dogs	3	10
Core, Legs	Squat	3	10
	Walking Lunge	3	10
	Side-to-side lunges	3	10

Core, Legs, Lower Back	Bridge (2 leg or 1 leg)	3	10
	Four-way Tap Drill (touch either side, top left, and top right)	3	10
Core, Arms, Shoulders	Push-Ups (any variety)	3	10
	Walk-Outs to push up position, hold-back to standing position	3	10
	Triceps Dips	3	10
	Mini Arm Circles (forward and backward)	3	30 sec.

*For more advanced training, seek the advice of a nationally registered strength and conditioning coach.

"THROWER'S TEN" WORKOUT PROGRAM

The "Thrower's Ten" program is a concise, upper extremity exercise regimen specifically designed for use by pitchers and throwers. Each exercise is designed to improve power, strength, and endurance of the shoulder and arm musculature. Throughout the baseball season, each exercise should be repeated ten to fifteen times, three to four times per week. Please note, however, this exercise program *should not* be used immediately before the start of a game or inning.

Tools needed:
- Stretch band or TheraBand
- 5-pound hand weight
- A fence or other stationary location
- Flat table

"Thrower's Ten Program Exercises"
- **Diagonal Patterns**
- **Diagonal Pattern D2 Extension:** Involved hand will grip tubing handle overhead and out to side. Pull tubing down and across your body to the opposite side of leg. During the motion, lead with your thumb.

- **Diagonal Pattern D2 Flexion:** Gripping tubing handle in hand of involved arm, begin with arm out from side 45 degrees and palm facing backward. After turning palm forward, proceed to flex elbow and bring arm up and over involved shoulder. Turn palm down and reverse to take arm to starting position.

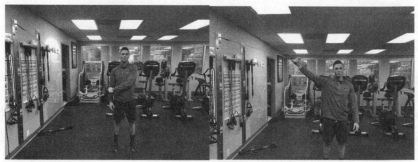

Figure 13.6

- **External and Internal Rotators**
- **External rotation at 0 degrees' abduction:** Stand with involved elbow fixed at side, elbow at 90 degrees, and involved arm across front of body. Grip tubing handle while the other end of tubing is fixed. Pull out arm, keeping elbow at side. Return tubing slowly and in control.
- **Internal rotation at 0 degrees' abduction:** Standing with elbow at side fixed at 90 degrees and shoulder rotated out, grip tubing handle while other end of tubing is fixed. Pull arm across body, keeping elbow at side. Return tubing slowly and in control.
- **External rotation at 90 degrees' abduction:** Stand with shoulder abducted to 90 degrees. Grip tubing handle while the other end is fixed straight ahead, slightly lower than the shoulder. Keeping shoulder abducted, rotate shoulder back, keeping elbow at 90 degrees. Return tubing and hand to start position. (Can be performed at slow and fast speed.)

- **Internal rotation at 90 degrees' abduction:** Stand with shoulder abducted to 90 degrees, externally rotated 90 degrees and elbow bent to 90 degrees. Keeping shoulder abducted, rotate shoulder forward, keeping elbow bent at 90 degrees. Return tubing and hand to start position. (Can be performed at slow and fast speed.)

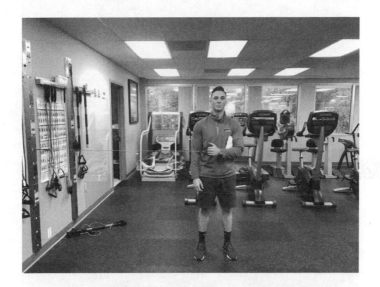

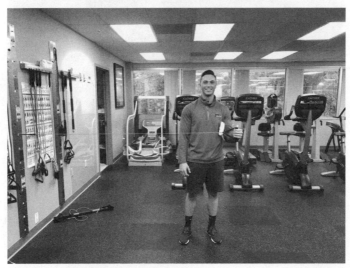

Figure 13.7

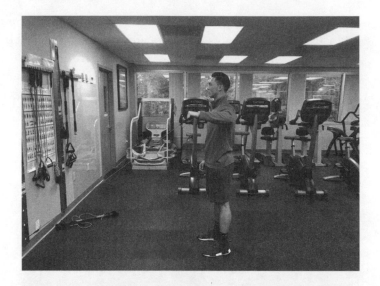

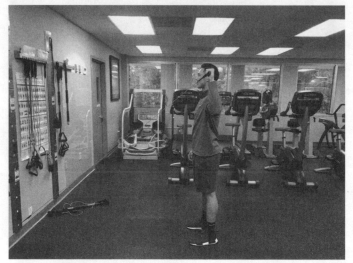

Figure 13.8

- **Shoulder abduction to 90 degrees:** Stand with arm at side, elbow straight and palm against side. Raise arm to the side, palm down, until arm reaches 90 degrees (shoulder level).

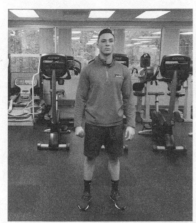
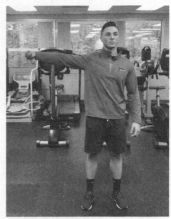

Figure 13.9

- **Scaption, External Rotation:** Stand with elbow straight and thumb up. Raise arm to shoulder level at 30-degree angle in front of body. Do not go above shoulder height. Hold two seconds and lower slowly.

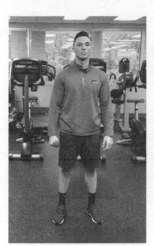
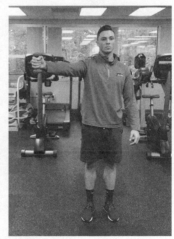

Figure 13.10

- **Side-Lying External Rotation:** Lie on uninvolved side, with involved arm at side of body and elbow bent to 90 degrees. Keeping the elbow of involved arm fixed to side, raise arm. Hold two seconds and lower slowly.

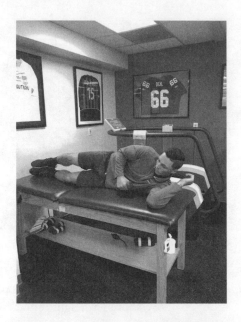

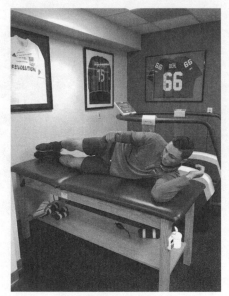

Figure 13.11

- **Prone Exercises**
- **Prone Horizontal Abduction (Neutral):** Lie on table, face down, with involved arm hanging straight to the floor and palm facing

down. Raise arm out to the side, parallel to the floor. Hold two seconds and lower slowly.

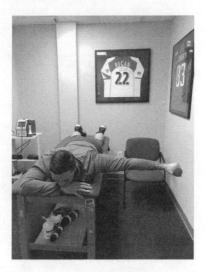

Figure 13.12

- **Prone Horizontal Abduction (Full ER, 100 degrees ABD):** Lie on table face down, with involved arm hanging straight to the floor and thumb rotated up (thumbs up). Raise arm out to the side with arm slightly in front of shoulder, parallel to the floor. Hold two seconds and lower slowly.

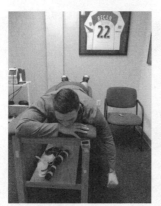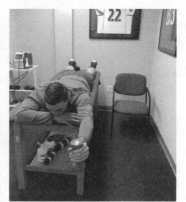

Figure 13.13

- **Prone Rowing:** Lying on your stomach with your involved arm hanging over the side of the table, dumbbell in hand and elbow straight. Slowly raise arm, bending elbow, and bring dumbbell as high as possible. Hold at the top for two seconds and slowly lower.

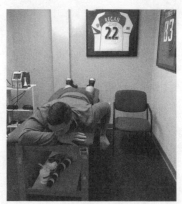

Figure 13.14

- **Prone Rowing into External Rotation:** Lying on your stomach with your involved arm hanging over the side of your table, dumbbell in hand and elbow straight. Slowly raise arm, bending elbow, up to the level of the table. Pause one second. Then rotate shoulder upward until dumbbell is even with the table, keeping elbow at 90 degrees. Hold at the top for two seconds, then slowly lower, taking two to three seconds.

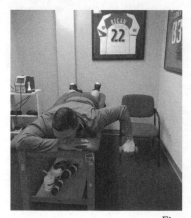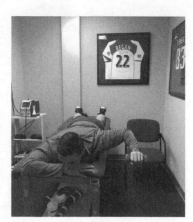

Figure 13.15

- **Press-ups:** Seated on a chair or table, place both hands firmly on the sides of the chair or table, palm down and fingers pointed outward. Hands should be placed equal with shoulders. Slowly push downward through the hands to elevate your body. Hold the elevated position for two seconds and lower body slowly.

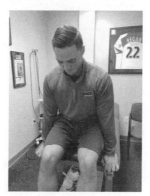
Figure 13.16

- **Push-ups:** Start in the down position with arms in a comfortable position. Place hands no more than shoulder width apart. Push up as high as possible, rolling shoulders forward after elbows are straight. Start with a push-up into wall. Gradually progress to a tabletop and eventually to the floor as tolerable.

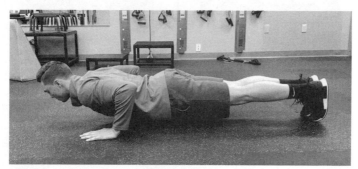
Figure 13.17

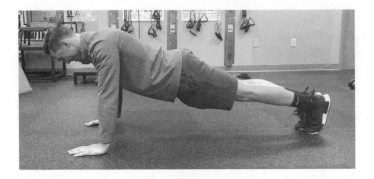

- **Elbow Flexion and Extension**
- **Elbow Flexion:** Standing with arm against side and palm facing inward, bend elbow upward, turning palm up as you progress.

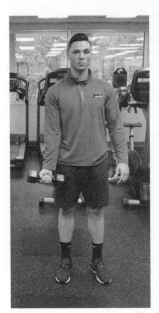 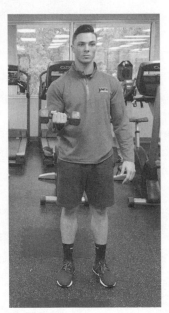

Figure 13.18

- **Elbow Extension (Abduction):** Raise involved arm overhead. Provide support at elbow from uninvolved hand. Straighten arm overhead. Hold two seconds and lower slowly.

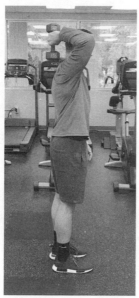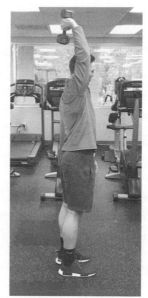

Figure 13.19

- **Wrist Exercises**
- **Wrist Extension:** Supporting the forearm (over biceps, above elbow) and, with palm facing downward, raise weight in hand as far as possible. Hold two seconds and lower slowly.

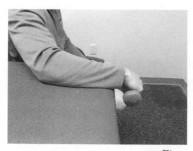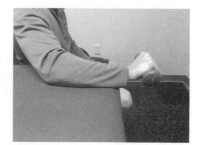

Figure 13.20

- **Wrist Flexion:** Supporting the forearm (over biceps, above elbow) and, with palm facing upward, lower a weight in hand as far as possible and then curl it up as high as possible. Hold for two seconds and then lower it slowly.

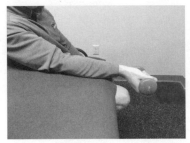 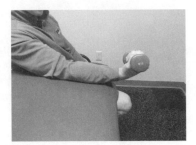

Figure 13.21

- **Supination:** Forearm supported on table with wrist in neutral position. Using a weight or hammer, roll wrist so palm is facing up. Hold for a two-count and return to starting position.

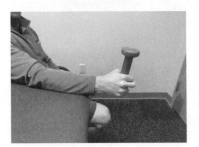 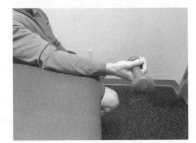

Figure 13.22

- **Pronation:** Forearm should be supported on a table with wrist in neutral position. Using a weight or a hammer, roll wrist so palm is facing down. Hold for a two-count and return to starting position.

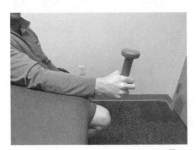 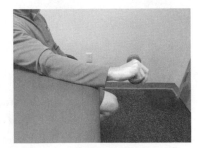

Figure 13.23

CHAPTER 14
by John Gallucci, Jr.

DEVELOPMENTAL TIMELINES: WHAT TO EXPECT FROM YOUR ATHLETE

Your six-year-old son or daughter is about to enter the sports world for the first time. It's their first day of practice and, naturally, you are very excited. The kid looks fantastic. The uniform is on, the cleats are all shined up, and you're heading to the field. So, as a parent, what should you expect?

Parents always wonder how good is little Johnny or Susie going to be? Will little Johnny or Susie be better than half the team? Will he or she be the best player? You'll realize very quickly on that first day of practice that little Johnny and Susie play just like everybody else. So you have to remember why you, as a parent, got your kids into athletics in the first place. It was to get them out with their friends, get them some exercise, and to teach them to play a sport. It wasn't to get them a college scholarship at six years old. It was, primarily, for them to have fun.

There are, however, certain things you can expect of your child athlete between the ages of six and ten from a physical, psychological, and social perspective. Let's take a look at some of those things.

Physical

If you compare five- and six-year-old boys and girls, they're not all the same size, they don't all weigh the same, and they don't all move the same. Their fingers and hands are different sizes. Everyone develops at a different pace, but, at that age, their fine motor skills—the coordination of small muscle movements, such as in the hands and fingers—are not yet developed. Even their gross motor skills—coordinated by larger muscle groups for full body movements such as walking and running—are still developing.

If you had those five- and six-year-olds line up in front of a tee and had them swing and hit the ball off the tee, you would see children who can't hit the ball at all, children who aren't sure whether they should stand on the left or right side, and children who hit the tee instead of the ball. And that's all okay. They're growing. So when you watch your child in that first day of practice, no matter the sport, you have to take a step back and understand and accept your child's developmental timeline.

During my son Charlie's fifth year, he could barely hold the tennis racquet. As he turned seven, I watched him hit the ball across the net with no problem. He also progressed to hitting forehands and backhands with no issues and was able to control the racket because his gross motor skills and his fine motor skills had caught up a bit with his body, which gave him more balance and stability, allowing him to actually play the sport appropriately. You, as a parent, will not believe how much your child will improve in a small time frame.

However, you can't rush them. You can't rush their growth, and you can't rush their muscles getting stronger or their bones growing. If your six-year-old son weighs 50 pounds and is in the 80th percentile, you can't make him jump to the 90th percentile. All you can possibly do is give your children good nutrition, make sure they exercise every day, support them, and make sure they are enjoying the activity. Honoring the developmental timeline is the most important thing.

If your son or daughter is low on the development chart, you should talk to your pediatrician and make sure it's okay for them to participate in organized sports. Most pediatricians will encourage it for muscular and skeletal development, since exercise makes the body stronger. When we try to protect our children because of their size or their weight, we limit them. If the child wants to play something, let them play. If your child has an interest, that's half the battle in athletics.

At this age, I encourage parents to let their children play multiple sports. This enables them to learn different elements of their body. They learn to use their balance and their muscles in different ways. In the long run, multisport athletes have a decreased risk of injuries. The variety helps to keep their interest, and, as they get older, they are more likely to stay involved with something that keeps them at some level of fitness.

Social Skills

The social integration of your child is essential to his or her development. I think it's very important for children from six to ten years old to socialize and interact with their peers. It's very important that parents don't select individual sports for their children at this age. Choose a team sport, such as baseball or softball, so your child can be in a social environment and have the opportunity to make friends. The sport will give them something in common and they'll want to go back to practice to see their friends. The friendships they develop will enrich the environment of the sport and help them learn the sport together and play the sport successfully.

Psychological Benefits

There are many parents who have never played a sport in their lives and are now introducing their children to sports. It's important to make sure the sport is about the child and his or her interests versus what sport you wanted to play or wish you could have played. So many kids today play the sports their parents push them toward.

Parents should never pressure children to perform beyond their capacity. It's counterproductive at best and dangerous at worst. Remember, your little athlete needs to develop an interest in the sport before he or she can truly compete. Criticism diminishes interest in playing, so don't hop on the negatives. For example, if your little baseball player can throw the ball really well, but has trouble hitting, you, as an adult, know he or she needs to work on hitting. Instead of pointing out their inability to hit the ball, motivate them to become better hitters. Make games out of it. You don't want to spend a lot of time on throwing because they're already good at it, but you do want to emphasize what a great job they're doing with throwing so they feel good about themselves and keep their interest in the sport.

Your support will enhance their interest in the game. Praise them when they do things well. Because there is a wide range of growth and maturation during the early stages, it's important to identify and reward the strengths of the less mature player.

What Should Practice Look Like?

A typical practice for the six- to ten-year-old athlete should be about an hour to an hour and ten minutes long. It should include a lot of different drills and activities to teach your child the sport, but it should, most importantly, be fun.

There are very few six- to ten-year-olds without a basic level of fitness. They can run for hours. So, at this age, a fitness component isn't really necessary. However, they should spend ten to fifteen minutes doing a low-level, basic warm-up and some stretching and flexibility work to give them a framework for how their practices will work as they mature in the sport. As they get older, the importance of a warm-up and flexibility will increase.

Then, the coach should actually have a teaching session, just as a teacher would have in a classroom. He or she should spend about twenty minutes working on a specific skill set, such as teaching a position or working on how to catch the ball.

Finally, the coach should give the kids twenty or thirty minutes to actually play the game, because that's when they're going to have the most fun, and you want them to have fun so they come running back to practice. Kids love to run, they love to score, and they love to be rewarded for doing well. The environment at this age needs to be very friendly, very educational, and very motivating to keep the children involved.

How Can You Help?

You have to remember that a parent-coach is exactly that: a parent who got home from work early that day and wants to coach his or her son or daughter. Some of them know nothing about the sport and are just really good people. Some of them know a little too much about the sport and think your six-year-old is going to land a full-time job in Major League Baseball. If your son or daughter has a coach who is a little over the top, you might need to talk to the coach and say, "Hey, listen, they're six years old. They're not getting paid a million dollars a year to hit the ball."

You have to make sure the child is learning the sport, is being encouraged, and is having a good time. So, if your son or daughter isn't getting all of that from the coach, you, as a parent, have to supplement.

The last thing you want is for your child to get to the next level and not understand how to play the game.

Have your child practice the skills he or she learns in practice at home for fifteen or twenty minutes a day so the coach doesn't have to use practice to reteach what was taught the last time. My son Charlie attended his first lacrosse camp when he was seven years old, where he learned how to throw and catch a lacrosse ball. At that camp, he threw really well but couldn't catch at all. His hand-eye coordination hadn't developed sufficiently for him to move the lacrosse stick quickly enough to catch it as the ball was coming to him.

When he returned from camp, we spent the next couple weeks practicing the skill at home. He had to catch and throw fifty times with his right hand and fifty with his left. To increase the fun element, we made a game out of it and rewarded him. If he was able to catch the ball twenty-five times, Charlie was rewarded with a half an hour of television. If he was able to catch more than twenty-five, he could choose a snack to enjoy while he watched television. Kids love rewards, so the motivation can really help them learn the sport.

WHAT TO EXPECT FROM YOUR ELEVEN- TO FOURTEEN-YEAR-OLD ATHLETE

Parents, do you remember when you hit puberty? Do you remember what you were going through? Understandably, you've probably chosen to forget. In these years, things are happening to your young athletes' bodies that they don't understand or recognize. They're going through physical, psychological, and hormonal changes. They're entering middle school and high school. Friends and peer groups become more involved. All these things can put massive stress on your child as he or she continues to develop physically, socially, and psychologically through athletics.

Physical Changes

Your child will have his or her biggest growth spurts during this time. Fine and gross motor skills will start to work better. This is when you start to perfect the minor skills, movements, and mechanics of the sport your child has chosen to play. They already know the rules and understand how to play the game, so now they can start to learn to do well at the game. From the ages of six to ten, they played many different positions to learn how the game worked. Now, they will start to hone in on one position. As pitchers, catchers, and infield or outfield players, they require different skill sets to play the game, and having increased fine motor skills will help them to hone those skills.

Once again, it's important to remember that all children grow at different rates. One twelve-year-old may weigh 95 pounds, while another is 150 pounds. Think about how the smaller child will feel when he or she is put on a baseball field with a much bigger child. He or she is going to feel he or she is at a competitive disadvantage due to size and strength. You have to be aware of those situations.

Social Skills

At this age, your children are changing schools, changing teachers, changing friends, and, possibly, changing neighborhoods if you relocate. Athletics help to meld everything together. Being on a sports team is your first introduction to a new area. My own daughter Stephanie was uprooted when we moved from New York to New Jersey. She knew no one in our new neighborhood or in her new high school but, as a freshman soccer player, she met other girls on the team before school started. The social implications and stresses of joining a new school were greatly reduced because, on the first day of class, she already knew people.

Keeping your son and daughter engaged with their peers is important. It gives them people to vent to who are going through the same things physically, socially, and psychologically. Being with their peers decreases their angst and anxiety. Adults: What's the one thing the doctor tells you when you have anxiety? He says to exercise. Your children need to exercise, because participating in sports will decrease their anxiety.

At this age, you also have to choose between school and club sports for your child. School sports give the opportunity to train and develop with children he or she already knows from his or her classes and is comfortable with. It's an opportunity for camaraderie and social interaction, and I think it's better for your son or daughter to be in a familiar environment. In club sports, the kids are from different towns and demographics, and, between the ages of eleven and fourteen, I don't think the kids are all psychologically developed enough to handle this advanced interaction. It can be overwhelming. Keeping a commonality is a little more enriching. Later on, the diversity of club sports can be enriching, as well, but, at this age, the home environment is very important.

Your child may be recruited by a private high school. As a parent, you have to decide based on what's best for your son or daughter. A scholarship is nice, but don't make the decision based solely on finances. What happens if your child isn't as good as the coach thought and doesn't make the team? What if your child gets hurt and can't play? What if he or she has to leave the school because you can't afford it without the athletic scholarship? You have to be prepared to handle that rejection and that situation. Send your child to a school that is within your means and will provide a good education. Sports, at this level, and at every level, are secondary.

Psychological Benefits

Peer pressure at this age is tremendous. Your child is consumed with what he or she is going to wear, what he or she looks like, and how many pimples he or she has. We all know teenagers can be a little moody, so you want to make sure that participating in sports puts your child in a good mood. They need to get some sort of psychological gratification from their sport. Simply put, they have to enjoy it.

Most parents start to pigeonhole children at this age into one specific sport, but that becomes repetitive. If children play the same position in the same sport all year long, it becomes tedious and they get bored. I believe it's important to be a multisport athlete, even at this level, not only for the physical benefits of being a diverse athlete, but also for the psychological reason of keeping their interest.

You want your child to want to be involved in different things. Studies show that, at thirteen years old, 70 percent of children in organized sports drop out of them because they've lost interest. Parents and coaches have to strive to keep them involved. To do that, sports have to be fun. At this age, there should not be a win-at-all-cost mentality. You want to have victories and the challenges of success but, psychologically, it still needs to be fun.

Playing Up

There certainly are fourteen-year-olds who are more talented than their peers. They have better motor skills and can dribble, skate, run, pass, throw, and score better than the other kids on their teams. We often advance those children to a higher level because we feel their skill level at the lower level was achieved easily. But you need to keep your children within their age group. If you advance your child too quickly at this time, you're going to force your child to work out and train with adults, which brings a new set of physical and psychological issues.

Here's an example. A fourteen-year-old boy, as a freshman in high school, weighs 180 pounds. Any football coach in America will say, "Holy cow, I can make this kid a beast over the next four years." He'll talk about scholarships and pro opportunities. But this boy is a freshman in high school. You don't know if he's going to play pro, or even play in college. No matter how big a child he is, the number one priority should always be development. Some states have enacted laws against playing freshman on the varsity team. In states that haven't, there are too many coaches who will take that fourteen-year-old, bring him up to varsity, and call it development, but then insert him into situations that can be detrimental to his health, not only physically, but mentally, as well.

That fourteen-year-old has growth plates in his bones that aren't developed and has stability issues because his gross motor skills are not as defined as a seventeen- or eighteen-year-old's. The younger child's musculoskeletal system is not developed enough to take a hit from a grown man whose growth plates are closed. Of course, a child can get hurt playing at his or her own age level, but it's different if two fourteen-year-olds are running into each other, rather than an eighteen-year-old running into a fourteen-year-old.

That fourteen-year-old will find himself laid up with a fractured growth plate and worrying whether his arm or leg will ever be normal. So, because the coach told you your child was ready for varsity sports, you're not sure if your child will ever play anything again. A fourteen-year-old child should not be playing against an eighteen-year-old man or woman.

There are psychological issues, as well. Do you want your thirteen-year-old son or daughter hanging out in the locker room and on the bus with an eighteen-year-old man or woman, talking about adult concepts like sexuality, drugs, and alcohol? Your child is still developing, and that's not the environment to do it in.

We pick good schools and good coaches so our children can develop in a good environment with their peers. I'm not saying you can't take the opportunity to train a year ahead. But when you jump two or three levels, it's usually a recipe for disaster. The last thing you want to do is have your preteen or early teenage son or daughter start to ask you questions about the social elements of an eighteen-year-old's life. Our goal is to keep our children training within their age group. You can get increased work and conditioning with a trainer in the sport to challenge your son or daughter, but to have them playing up levels is not such a great idea.

Growth Plates

Just because your child is big doesn't mean his or her bones are any more mature. Bone growth is dictated by hormonal and age values, not size. There are kids at fourteen, fifteen, or sixteen whose growth plates are closed. But, in the majority of kids that age, they are not.

Growth plates, or physes, are zones of cartilage at the end of each long bone, such as the tibia or femur. These bones grow due to contributions of new bone from the growth plate. Because the cartilage is soft, it is particularly vulnerable to injury as a child develops. Growth plates are so fragile that an injury that results in a joint sprain in an adult can result in growth-plate fracture in a child. These fractures require immediate medical attention to prevent the fractured bone from healing improperly by growing crooked or shorter than the opposite limb.

What Should Practice Look Like?

As younger children, your little athletes learned the fundamentals of the game. Now, as they begin to gravitate toward a specific position on the field—e.g., defense, offense, infield, or outfield—they can begin to learn the fundamentals of the specific position and the skill set necessary for that position. However, their training should still involve a sense of play to keep their interest, especially because the duration of the practice will likely increase to what should be a fun, regimented, and involved two hours, three to four times a week.

As always, there should be a warm-up and stretch session for ten to fifteen minutes. Practice should then progress to work on skill development for their position (i.e., pitchers and catchers) and position development on the field as a group for about thirty minutes (i.e., fielding grounders and pop-ups). Then, they should practice live game situations for another thirty minutes. For example, in baseball, the coach may call out a game situation, and the team as a whole has to work through the play. There should then be a fifteen- to twenty-minute fitness component. It doesn't need to be cardio if they've already been running or skating around for most of the practice. It can, for example, focus on core strength, because, in sports such as hockey, soccer, baseball, lacrosse, field hockey, and golf, a strong core is necessary to reduce the rotary forces generated by the movements of the sport and decrease the incidence of injury. Finally, there should be a cooldown and stretch.

Coaches at this level are still youth development coaches. But is it a parent? Is it as someone who was good at the sport at one time? Is it someone who is running an academy and who is making money? You need to pick a coach or club that errs on the side of developing your child's skill, strength, conditioning, and positioning in the sport, but, at this level, coaches also need to understand and be equipped to deal with emotional twelve-, thirteen-, and fourteen-year-olds.

The Offseason

At many high schools across the country, seasons begin with several days to a week of double-session practices. But please understand this: You cannot condition a child in three days. You can't take a child who did nothing all fall or winter, bring him or her in on March 1, and expect them, for multiple days in a row, to break down muscle and work their tails off cardiovascularly with no time to regenerate and recoup. They're all going to wind up at the doctor or with the physical therapist or the athletic trainer.

I'm not saying they can't practice twice a day. The practices just need to involve as much strategic practice as physical practice so the athletes have time to recover. Teach them to understand the game plan. What are we doing? What plays are we running? If this happens, you move this way. This is what happens when a ground ball is hit to second with a player on third. All of that is fine. You just can't condition morning and night and expect peak performance. All you get when you overwork is a tired team that isn't ready to practice the next day. This is why your child needs to be on a year-long conditioning program. We know physiologically it takes six weeks to develop muscle. Even professional athletes have gotten smart enough that most of their preseasons are six weeks long, but their conditioning is year-round. We do it in the pros, we do it in the colleges, so why aren't we doing it for our youth? If a pro athlete can't be ready in just one week, how can we expect that of a seventh grader?

Another way to keep your child conditioned is to encourage participation in multiple sports. Keep in mind, though, that even if your child plays football in the fall and baseball in the spring, he still needs to condition in the winter and summer to keep his body prepared.

How Can Parents Help?

Parents should be very involved in the skill set. Look at the position your child is going to play and make sure he or she practices the skill set of that position. Make sure they are well-conditioned and have proper biomechanics and equipment for their sport so they'll stay out of the doctor's office and the PT clinic. Most athletic trainers can assess the biomechanics of running, jumping, and throwing, but there are also outside coaches who can ensure your child is moving efficiently and correctly, which is essential to remaining injury-free. As a parent, you also have to implement good nutrition and hydration protocols, which were discussed in Chapter 10.

WHAT TO EXPECT FROM YOUR FIFTEEN- TO EIGHTEEN-YEAR-OLD ATHLETE

Between the ages of fifteen and eighteen, your child's participation in athletics becomes more gratifying, more goal- and career-oriented, more targeted, and more sport-specific. Depending on your child's skill level, it can also become college-specific, and that's great. To get ahead in college is, really, to get ahead professionally.

Physical Considerations

Your child's musculoskeletal maturity is now coming into an adult form. They have more muscular gains at this point. Their growth plates are starting to close. They have a better depth of understanding of their fine motor skills. Children can start to focus on fine-tuning their skills in their sport because their gross and fine motor skills are really in tune, and their entire body is now mature. At this level, you see more training regimens being implemented, which include strength and conditioning components off the court or field.

Because children in this age group focus more on one sport, you have to worry about the possibility of increased overuse injuries because of the repetitiveness involved in playing one sport year-round.

Social Skills

Your children have very complex social lives at this age, which adds to their everyday stress. They start to date, so they're always worried: Is my boyfriend or girlfriend mad at me? Am I accepted by my peers? Am I going out with ten of my friends or am I not going out at all? Do I have to go to work? Should I go for a run or go to the movies and eat five pounds of popcorn? Have I done my homework? Have I studied for my anatomy test?

Your children have more responsibilities than ever and time management comes into play. But there is no better forum than athletics to teach your child leadership qualities and organization. Your children get life lessons while playing organized sports. Of course, we want them to be involved for the fitness component of staying healthy and the social component of having friends, but athletics also teach our kids to become mature, responsible adults by putting them into situations with coaches, referees, and teammates that will teach them to be respectful, diplomatic, and responsible. Sports can help prepare your son or daughter for life.

Psychological Benefits

Your children are starting to make more decisions for themselves and for their future. Their work ethic is evolving, and they have more of an interest in what they're doing. They give up the multitude of sports and focus on the sports in which they excel.

They start to understand what stress is. Are my grades good enough to get into school? Do I have to get a part-time job to support myself or to help support the household?

Peer pressure is tremendous. Is your son or daughter opening up and talking to someone? Is there someone they can vent to? Are you constantly on them, adding more stress? Teachers will get mad at me for this, but it's not a bad idea to keep your son or daughter home from school and have a fun day of relaxation. Some of the best coaches take a day off to detox their teams in the middle of the playoffs. You need that. In youth athletics, why can't we also take a day to take a step back?

What Should Practice Look Like?

Most athletes at the high school or club sport level have training five days a week for two to two and a half hours. Most coaches will structure the practice similarly to the practices for the younger ages. There should be a warm-up for ten to fifteen minutes, with a dynamic or static stretch depending on the coach's philosophies. There should be twenty to thirty minutes of skill development to fine-tune the skills of the athletes at their particular positions.

At this level, the attention span is better and the athletes understand the game better, so they can do more repetitions without fatigue or distraction. Team concepts should then be worked on for twenty to thirty minutes. They'll walk through situations to understand in what position they're supposed to be based on what play is being run or what scenario they're in and how it works. The kids are more developed mentally and can handle this. Then the coach will move into situation play for twenty to thirty minutes, putting the athletes in an offensive or defensive situation and have them play it out. Coaches will probably do less full scrimmaging at this age, but will let the team go live for twenty or thirty minutes because it's both beneficial and fun. There will almost always be a fitness component toward the end of practice for fifteen to thirty minutes that will include both an aerobic and strength component, followed by a cooldown and stretch.

A Few Words about Strength and Conditioning

The phrase "strength and conditioning" is a term used to describe any athletic training done outside the realm of one's sport and designed to make an athlete more physically fit for the demands of his or her sport.

As a parent, you must take note of what your child is doing on the strength and conditioning front, as different modalities can cause repetition and overuse injuries.

Is My Athlete College-Bound?

Applying to colleges and getting accepted to a college of their choice provides additional pressures for athletes in this age category, and there are a lot of decisions that you and your child must make together at this point. Do I want to play sports in college? Do I need or want a scholarship? Am I being offered a scholarship? Am I good enough to get a scholarship?

As a parent, you need to have realistic expectations of your child. Is he or she talented compared to the other players on his or her youth team? How does that compare to the county, the state, and the nation? If your child is the No. 2 player on the township baseball team, that's fantastic, but that doesn't mean he or she has what it takes to be in the national pool or to get a college scholarship. If your child plays at a high level and college coaches are calling you, your child has the talent required to be a collegiate athlete. If you're out banging on doors continually, trying to tell everyone how good your child is, he or she probably doesn't have the talent. If they're good enough, people will find them and make sure they have the opportunity to play. You can be an advocate, yes, but you don't want to be a fool. If you're unsure about how to proceed with regard to college athletics, speak to your child's coach or your high school athletic director.

CHAPTER 15
by Dr. Christopher Ahmad

LITTLE LEAGUER'S ELBOW

Most people in baseball have heard the term "Little Leaguer's Elbow" but don't understand what it truly is. Little Leaguer's Elbow is a term first coined in 1960 that describes a condition caused by repetitive throwing motions, especially in children who play sports that involve throwing. The pitching motion that causes a valgus stress to the inside elbow joint is resisted by the UCL. The UCL is attached to the bone in a location that includes a growth plate called the medial apophysis. This is also the location where the forearm muscles attach, which adds additional stress to the growth plate. The growth plate is intrinsically weaker than adult bone that has matured and stopped growing. For kids, the growth plate is the weak link in the chain. Adult pitchers do not experience the same injury because they do not have the relatively weak open growth plate in the elbow. Instead, a more common injury in adult athletes is direct injury to the UCL, an injury that often requires Tommy John surgery for the athlete to resume high-level competitive throwing.

My clinical assistants often perform a very brief history for patients who present to my office for evaluation of their elbow pain. They obtain the patient's demographic information, such as what sport they play, how many teams they play on, what position they play, and what and where it hurts and for how long. Sometimes, the most important piece of information is what the patient's age is. If the patient's age is between twelve and fourteen, the sport is baseball, and the location of pain is the elbow, the issue is most likely to be a condition called Little Leaguer's Elbow.

There is a very unique situation where there is an overlap between a young athlete who's developing increased height/weight/body mass and strength with increasing throwing velocity. This overlaps with persistent skeletal growth in the growing child. The area where the bone grows is weaker than tendons and ligaments; therefore, the twelve- to fourteen-year-old has a perfect window where he or she is throwing harder and generating more force on the elbow, but the elbow is still vulnerable at the growth plate and becomes injured.

Signs and Symptoms of Little Leaguer's Elbow

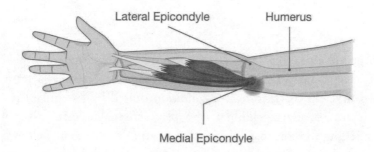

Patients often present to the office for evaluation of pain because it stops their ability to play. They explain that they've been throwing and, after some detective work, I usually discover a history of excessive throwing and a sense that the throwing is becoming harder with more velocity. The patient can easily point to the location of pain on the inside part of the elbow. It only hurts with throwing and, typically, doesn't hurt with routine activities such as carrying books, or other activities such as homework. The examination is specific for two things: There is usually no ecchymosis or bruising and swelling, and no limitations in motion, but there's simply direct tenderness when pushing on the area of bone at the growth plate and pain when stressing the elbow that puts tension on the growth plate. X-rays reveal that the area of growth plate, which is usually one to two mm in thickness, is increased in size and may be double the normal width. MRI scans are usually not necessary as the diagnosis is made simply from the history, physical exam, and X-rays.

How to Treat Little Leaguer's Elbow

Treatment can be frustrating for the player, the family, coaches, and even for the doctor. The treatment is to stop throwing for four to six weeks while working on core and leg strengthening, and shoulder and elbow strengthening. Then, at four to six weeks, if the examination shows a return to normal, a progressive throwing program with optimized throwing mechanics is initiated. It can be an additional six weeks before the athlete can be game-ready; therefore, the treatment can take three months and, unfortunately, in some situations, well over nine months, and sometimes even twelve.

In some situations, although it's much less common than standard Little Leaguer's Elbow, the growth plate bone can actually be ripped off and fractured from the attachment site. The muscles, which also attach to the bone, tend to displace the fractured bone. If this occurs, then it creates an instability problem at the elbow where getting back to throwing can be very challenging without pain. In addition, there are situations where the bone may actually not heal, and that, also, can be a very painful situation and a difficult surgical challenge. Therefore, if the bone is fractured, surgery is recommended. The bone is put back to its normal position and fixed with a screw that holds it in place while it heals and allows early and aggressive range of motion.

While doing end-of-season physicals with the Yankees one year, I met a professional baseball player on the pitching staff who had a normal elbow exam, but did have a scar on the inside aspect of his elbow. When I palpated his elbow, I could feel the contour of a screw below the skin and in his bone where the growth plate once existed. I asked him how old he was when he fractured his growth plate, and he said, "Thirteen."

Unfortunately, once or twice a year, I take care of a throwing athlete who had a fracture of this growth plate that was not treated surgically and failed to heal on its own. To correct this unhealed bone fracture, I have to surgically remove extensive scar tissue to get the bone fragment back into its normal position. The bone fragment is often deformed and fragile and requires a delicate balance of placing forceful screws to ensure it heals while avoiding too much screw pressure that will simply crush and fragment the bone.

CHAPTER 16
by Dr. Christopher Ahmad

CAPITELLAR OSTEOCHONDRITIS DISSECANS (OCD)

As discussed in Chapter 1, throwing athletes, especially those who haven't hit puberty yet, experience unique forces on their elbows. The inside part of the elbow has a pulling or tension force that stresses the ligament and can cause problems with the growth plate and the ligament. The outside aspect of the elbow gets compressive forces with repetitive throwing. It's as if the outside of the elbow is getting pounded like a hammer hitting a nail. The area of bone most vulnerable to injury is called the capitellum. The capitellum is round and the size of a grape. The overlying cartilage is usually healthy, but the bone that supports this cartilage underneath often has limited blood supply. Therefore, the pounding on this bone caused by throwing can create small microscopic injuries to the bone and, because the bone has poor blood supply, it does not heal well. The consequence is that the bone injury progresses and the bone becomes weak and unable to support the overlying cartilage. If the cartilage, which is now unsupported by bone, then becomes fragmented or loose, it can create mechanical locking and catching in the elbow. This condition is unique to young throwers, but can also affect athletes such as gymnasts who have repetitive forces across the elbow. I hope this book helps parents and coaches recognize the importance in having young throwers assessed by a sports specialist if having elbow pain and, especially, if they have a sensation of locking (their elbow getting stuck).

Signs and Symptoms

Athletes with capitellar OCD often present because of an inability to throw, and with a distinctive and uncomfortable locking or catching sensation. Young patients will explain that they have the sensation that a small object similar to a marble is floating in the elbow and, at times, the marble gets stuck where they then become unable to flex or extend their elbow. The examination by the physician typically reveals decreased ability to extend the elbow fully and tenderness over the outside part of the elbow. Swelling may or may not be present. X-rays may demonstrate the appearance of loose pieces of bone or decreased bone density in the area of the capitellum, but often, X-rays are normal. An MRI scan is most useful to determine the existence of capitellar OCD. In addition, an MRI can grade the lesion as being either intact, partially detached, or, in some situations, an entire fragment of detached cartilage. Accurate and early diagnosis with an MRI allows for earlier intervention and treatment. Unrecognized OCD lesions can progress in size and damage to the joint and have less ability to heal, or even less ability to be corrected with surgery.

How to Treat Capitellar OCD

The treatment for capitellar OCD is dictated by patient age, activity level, and size and stability of the lesion. Intact lesions in young patients are most commonly treated with a period of rest, often with an elbow brace. Physical therapy is employed to help with swelling and restoration of motion and strength in the elbow, the shoulder, leg, and core muscles. When examination shows a return to normal, typically at six to twelve weeks, then a progressive throwing program can be initiated using proper throwing mechanics. These athletes need to be closely observed to avoid a recurrence of symptoms or progression in the stage of the lesion. For example, if the athlete throws with continued pain, it suggests the lesion is not healed well and can progress to becoming loose or unstable, which greatly changes prognosis.

If the fragment is either partially or fully separated, then surgery is required, especially in an older patient who wishes to stay active. Surgery is performed arthroscopically, which requires inserting a camera into the elbow joint. The arthroscope is then used to examine the entire elbow, looking for any loose pieces or fragments, which are identified or removed. The focus of the surgery is then directed to inspection of the capitellum where the defect or the lesion exists. This is the source of the loose floating fragments. The defect, if small, can be treated with a technique to create a "healing response." Perforations are made in the bone with small pins that cause bleeding from the bone that eventually creates scar tissue, also called fibrocartilage, that fills the defect. Following surgery, the postoperative course requires protection for two to three weeks with an elbow brace. Physical therapy is performed to regain range of motion and strengthening of the elbow, shoulder, core, and leg muscles—the whole kinetic chain. More aggressive strengthening occurs at three months, and throwing programs can be initiated somewhere between four and five months. Full participation in sports typically requires up to six months.

Occasionally, drilling or microfracture treatment is inadequate to treat larger lesions. Treatment is better with a grafting technique called osteochondral grafting. This procedure requires taking bone and cartilage plugs from cadavers or people who have donated their tissue and inserting it into the defect of the capitellum. This can be done either with the arthroscope or through an open technique with an incision. The goal is to restore the normal contour of the capitellum. The advantage of this technique is that the healing will be more consistent with normal cartilage rather than scar tissue cartilage. However, this surgical technique is challenging and requires an experienced surgeon. I recently studied this on cadaver elbows and demonstrated the ability to perform this procedure with precision using the arthroscope.

The ability to return to baseball with proper treatment of capitellar OCD is encouraging. While some injuries can be predictable, cartilage injuries are not. Therefore, capitellar OCD lesions, if suspected, should be evaluated, and proper treatment initiated as soon as possible to limit the progression, have more predictable healing, and return to sport.

There seems to be a familial inheritance with this condition. I have treated families with siblings all having capitellar OCD. One family I treated included a baseball player and his sister, a gymnast, both with capitellar OCD. The baseball player made a full recovery with arthroscopic treatment in his throwing arm. The gymnast developed pain and similar symptoms in her right elbow and was found to have capitellar OCD and required surgery. After a full recovery and return to gymnastics, she then developed capitellar OCD in the left elbow. Amongst the two kids, there were three surgeries. Thankfully, they're both continuing in their sports at this time.

CHAPTER 17
by Dr. Christopher Ahmad

YOUTH ELBOW INJURIES, FRACTURES, AND AVULSIONS

Several injuries are specific to young athletes. They live with a unique set of circumstances where their growth plates are still open and vulnerable to injury, but the athlete is growing to a size and strength where the magnitude of force generated at the elbow is large enough to cause injury. Especially in the setting of increased specialization, year-round playing, and lack of rest periods, injuries to the growth plates on the inside of the elbow are becoming increasingly common. In some situations, the growth plate can completely fracture and move several centimeters out of its normal position. In addition, injuries to the UCL itself, which was a rare occurrence in a young athlete, are becoming more prevalent.

Signs and Symptoms of Fractures of the Elbow

Patients with the medial epicondyle avulsion fracture complain of a discrete event when throwing a ball hard had a sudden onset of acute pain. They often get swelling and bruising along the inside of their elbow. Examination reveals tenderness over the medial elbow, along with pain with stress testing. X-rays often confirm the diagnosis, and, occasionally, CT scans or MRI scans are used to identify associated injuries or the degree of displacement or movement of the stress fracture.

How to Treat Elbow Fractures

The general population of non-throwing athletes can be managed well, inoperatively, with a period of mobilization, followed by rehabilitation. These patients often injure their medial epicondyle from a fall or even an elbow dislocation. However, for the throwing athlete, displacement can result in continued pain, failure of the bone to heal, pain, and instability. Some surgeons recommend surgical treatment for very small levels of displacement up to 2 to 5 mm. Often, surgery has the most predictable result with faster rehabilitation.

Operative treatment includes an incision over the inside aspect of the elbow and reducing the fracture by fixing it with a screw. This allows immediate range-of-motion exercises with predictable and accelerated healing, compared to non-operative treatment. And, while it's unusual, there is at least one Yankee pitcher who had this injury as a young thrower in adolescence and who is now playing at the professional level.

The other ligament attachment to the ulnar bone is called the sublime tubercle. Stress from repetitive throwing can cause an injury here. The ligament is stronger than the bone and may be prone to avulsion-type fracture. Patient complaints are similar to the proximal avulsion fracture with a sudden onset of pain and swelling, and even ecchymosis. X-rays often make the diagnosis, but it may require an MRI or CT scan. For fractures that are in a good position and have not moved, treatment includes a period of elbow rest with the elbow immobilized in a brace. After the bone heals as observed on X-rays, the treatment then includes restoration of elbow range of motion and strength. For those patients who fail non-operative treatment where the fracture simply does not heal, or is displaced, surgery is performed. This requires open dissection of the fracture and fixation of the bone with strong screws.

UCL INJURY

UCL injuries in the young growing population were previously thought to be relatively rare. Often, these injuries occur when the patient is older because the growth plate is so much weaker than the ligament. However, as more athletes play at higher levels with increased stress, we are seeing more UCL injuries.

Signs and Symptoms of UCL Injury

Young athletes who throw typically complain of pain during the late cocking acceleration phases of throwing, localized to the inside aspect of their elbow. They can suffer loss of velocity and accuracy. Physical examination is consistent with tenderness over the ulnar collateral ligament and pain with stress testing. An MRI scan is usually diagnostic. A careful assessment of associated injuries is performed, including flexor pronator mass avulsions and ulnar neuritis.

Ideal treatment for a young patient is non-operative. General considerations that also affect treatment decisions include the patient's level of competition, age, position, and prior treatments or episodes of pain. The injury may be characterized as complete, partial, or a sprain of the ligament.

Grade One lesions, or those with fluid or edema in the surrounding ligament, is a ligament that is essentially swollen from a sprain.

Grade Two lesions display partial disruption of the ligament with ligament fibers torn, but some fibers remain intact.

Grade Three lesions are complete tears where no ligament fibers are intact.

Initial treatment of Grade One or Two UCL tears involves a period of rest, anti-inflammatory medication, and a progressive strengthening program, including the flexor pronator, mass rotator cuff, core, and legs. After approximately three months, a progressive throwing program with proper pitching mechanics is initiated.

A recent treatment option that has gained popularity in my practice is the use of platelet-rich plasma. This strategy uses the growth factors related to an individual patient by taking his or her blood, spinning it in a centrifuge, isolating the growth factors, and injecting it in the area of UCL injury under ultrasound guidance.

For young patients, a treatment option that is not as popular with older patients is primary repair. For younger patients with symptomatic UCL tears, primary repair is appealing because the ligament may not have undergone global injury patterns, and overall quality may be good. In addition, the younger athletes may have better healing potential, and their future career in throwing sports is not as clear.

Previously, this procedure was done with a simple suturing of the injured part of the ligament. More recently, an internal brace technique has been employed. I have experience with this internal brace where the ligament is repaired and, to protect the repair, a high-tensile suture tape is fixed on both ends, protecting the ligament repair. This greatly accelerates the overall recovery process. Players with a repair and an internal brace when compared to a standard Tommy John ligament reconstruction may be able to achieve their return to play in up to six months, which is typically half the time of the standard Tommy John surgery.

CHAPTER 18
by Dr. Christopher Ahmad

ELBOW STRESS REACTION AND STRESS FRACTURES

Stress fractures involving the elbow have become increasingly common in baseball players. In addition, stress reactions that, ten years ago, were not well recognized, have now become commonplace. Baseball players are uniquely susceptible to stress reactions and stress fractures. Our knowledge of stress fractures mostly derives from the more usual locations of lower extremity stress fractures, most commonly related to the impact of running and jumping. For the thrower, stress reactions are primarily related to the repetitive, unique, and enormous forces from throwing.

Bone is extremely dynamic and undergoes bone formation and resorption according to the stress placed on it. Appropriate loading or stress to bone is healthy and creates strong bones. Too little, or excessive, loading can create injury. Abnormal or pathologic changes in bone can occur when more bone resorption occurs rather than bone formation in areas of increased stress. Olecranon stress reaction or fracture is the most common bone injury that causes pain in baseball players. The stress on the back elbow bone occurs from rapid elbow extension forces from throwing, or in the lead arm when hitting. In addition, stress to the ulna can be increased in the setting of ulnar collateral ligament deficiency. Therefore, some patients will have combined injuries of olecranon stress and UCL tears.

Signs and Symptoms of Stress Related Injury

A sudden increase in the amount of throwing can cause stress injury-related elbow pain. A position player who suddenly becomes a pitcher and throws right-handed and bats left-handed (right elbow is the lead elbow) can put an overwhelming rapid increase in stress to the olecranon bone. Pain occurs in the deceleration phase of throwing where players describe it as pain after the ball is released. A physical exam will demonstrate decreased range of motion and tenderness over the olecranon bone. There will also be pain when forcibly extending the elbow. The differential diagnosis is related to bone spurs or loose bodies in the back part of the elbow.

Plain X-rays are sensitive to picking up an advanced stage stress fracture. However, stress reactions or more mild forms of stress fracture require an MRI scan. Unfortunately, MRI scans often do not accurately demonstrate the extent of the pathology. This is one of the few areas where additional study via a CT scan, which visualizes bone very well, is necessary for the diagnosis.

Young throwers have a growth plate at the area of triceps insertion called an apophysis, which is well visualized on X-rays as children reach age nine to eleven. The growth plate in this area fuses at age fifteen to seventeen. A unique injury can occur in this young adolescent patient where the growth plate does not normally go on to fuse due to the stresses of throwing. In essence, this condition is a stress injury or stress fracture to the olecranon growth plate.

How to Treat Stress Reactions

For athletes younger than thirteen years old, rest, use of a brace, and avoiding extension and throwing often facilitates healing. If non-operative treatment fails to heal the injury with time, then surgery is indicated. For athletes between fourteen and sixteen, early operative management is typically necessary to fix an olecranon stress growth plate injury. This is most often achieved with screws placed across the fracture site to achieve compression.

Mature baseball players who are no longer growing who develop a significant olecranon stress fracture often require surgery. For less severe injuries, an attempt at non-operative treatment with a period of rest, a brace, and a bone stimulator can be used. However, seasonal and career timing may warrant earlier surgical intervention to have predictable healing and avoid further lost time from occurring if non-operative treatment is attempted and fails. The surgical treatment, typically, requires that screws be placed across the stress fracture to compress the fracture and force the healing process to occur. Stress fractures can be in different locations and orientations, and the screw configuration is based on the given fracture characteristics. Some very small stress fractures at the tip can be treated with arthroscopic surgery to remove the small area of fractured olecranon tip that often includes a bone spur on the stress fracture, which is also removed.

OLECRANON STRESS REACTION

In this situation, a stress fracture has not occurred, but the bone is reacting to the increased force in what's termed "the stress reaction." MRI scans will show high-intensity signal in the bone. It's similar to a signal that would occur from getting a bruise to the bone from a direct blow, such as getting hit by a pitch. Treatment is non-operative, consisting of six weeks of rest with a brace to limit full elbow extension, followed by a progressive strengthening program. At twelve weeks, a throwing program with emphasis on proper throwing mechanics is started. Often, a bone growth stimulator is recommended to enhance the healing.

In summary, olecranon stress fractures and stress reactions are likely secondary to the unique complex interactions that the elbow joint bones and ligaments undergo in the setting of rapid, increased throwing volume and intensity. Clinical suspicion of olecranon stress fractures should remain high, and it's often undiagnosed for too long a time. Imaging, including a CT scan, is necessary to rule out a stress fracture. An MRI is extremely sensitive for stress reaction. Surgery is very successful in healing the fracture, alleviating symptoms, and allowing return to play.

CHAPTER 19
by Dr. Christopher Ahmad

MAKING TOMMY JOHN SURGERY HISTORY

I participated in a panel discussion in 2015 with James Andrews, and we discussed the fact that, if you take a sufficiently careful history when confronted with a Tommy John injury in a professional athlete, you will find that 50 to 60 percent of the players first had some elbow problems between the ages of twelve and fourteen. The importance of arm health at young ages is paramount and can certainly affect an athlete's high school, collegiate, and/or professional career. Making Tommy John surgery history must begin with arm health early in athletes' athletic development so they can enjoy an injury-free future.

The strategy for prevention is education, guidelines to avoid overuse/abuse, and premature professionalism, as well as correcting the misperceptions of baseball elbow injuries. The throwing athlete, more than any other athlete, has a complementary group of stakeholders to assist him or her—parents, coaches, physical therapists, orthopedic surgeons, sports medicine specialists, strength and conditioning coaches, nutritionists, mental health coaches, and researchers. Everyone has the ability to have an effect.

Pitch Counts

Pitch counts are the purest and simplest way to manage overuse in baseball. In 2008, Little League Baseball implemented specific pitch count rules designed to ensure that youth pitchers got the proper amount of rest. These rules divided players into categories based on their age and the number of pitches thrown in a given day, mandating up to three full days of rest before taking the mound again. Many independent travel teams now have rules regarding pitch counts and set guidelines for limiting days of rest and the cumulative amount of pitching allowable. It is clear that young pitchers who throw more than eight months out of the year are more likely to sustain an injury. Therefore, in addition to pitch counts, a period of rest should be instituted, while pitching with arm fatigue should be avoided.

Pitch Count and Required Rest Limitations

Age	Daily Max (Pitches)	Required Rest (Pitches)	Required Rest (Pitches)	Required Rest (Pitches)	Required Rest (Pitches)	Required Rest (Pitches)
		0 Days	1 Day	2 Days	3 Days	4 Days
7-8	50*	1-20	21-35	36-50	N/A	N/A
9-10	75*	1-20	21-35	36-50	51-65	66+
11-12	85*	1-20	21-35	36-50	51-65	66+
13-14	95*	1-20	21-35	36-50	51-65	66+
15-16	95*	1-30	31-45	46-60	61-75	76+
17-18	105*	1-30	31-45	46-60	61-75	76+

Source: USA Little League 2017

Pitchers should adhere to pitch counts and rest and avoid playing on multiple teams. If a pitcher is supposed to rest, he or she should not go to another team and pitch. Additionally, baseball players should be encouraged to play multiple positions. This decreases the likelihood of injury and enhances performance by improving understanding of the strategy behind each position in order to develop different skills. Playing another position has to be factored into their throwing volume. It avoids overworking one set of muscles or joints to the point of injury.

The catcher is another important position with high throwing volume, with the second highest risk of injury related to overuse. Encouraging players to rotate through different positions helps to rest certain muscle groups.

NEW TECHNOLOGY SUPPORTS PITCH MANAGEMENT

Adding to the complexity of the Tommy John epidemic is the lack of easily accessible data at the youth level. Games are recorded far less consistently and meticulously than college or professional games, leaving no hard track record. Mobile device apps are now available to help coaches and parents more accurately track pitch counts, which can be tracked across different teams, enabling them to better protect young arms from overuse.

FUNCTIONAL ASSESSMENT AND BIOMECHANICS

Research devices that provide biomechanical assessment were once just that: research devices. Now, sophisticated biomechanical assessment can be used in individual young athletes and mature and professional athletes for injury risk assessment, using video analysis systems. The tests screen for muscle imbalances, muscle weakness, and inflexibility in specified movements that are predictive of injury. Once risk is identified, a corrective program can be implemented. Previously, these biomechanical analyses required heavy technologies with hours of testing and data analysis, but technology has now been streamlined in such a way that a whole baseball team can run through an injury risk assessment within an hour.

Many parents and coaches are more aware of the injury risk associated with the use of radar guns as a method of measuring performance. Radar guns now can be used as a device to monitor throws, give objective feedback on the throwing effort, and then have effort adjusted accordingly. This can help with bullpen sessions, for example, so that pitchers are throwing with guided effort. In fact, our research shows that throwing efforts are highly variable in young athletes when not monitored. Throwing distances are traditionally used as a guide to the effort of throwing. Throwing 120 feet requires more effort than throwing sixty feet, for example. However, some athletes will throw with too much effort at sixty feet as if to throw through the person they are throwing with. Therefore, distances are imprecise for managing throwing effort and optimal stress to the elbow and shoulder.

As more technology applications become available, they will help monitor workload fatigue and help us understand when an athlete requires a period of rest for tissue rejuvenation. Sleep apps, for example, and nutrition logs further enhance our ability to guide the growing athlete.

RESEARCH INITIATIVES WILL FURTHER IMPROVE PREVENTION AND TREATMENT

MLB formed a UCL research committee, which I serve on, with several research initiatives started each year. Every study is designed to investigate a variable believed to be involved in UCL injury. Research in this area is tedious and takes time before results are available to guide new prevention or treatment.

One of the more exciting projects is the initiative of a multicenter Tommy John injury registry. This allows any player who has Tommy John surgery at any given medical center around the country to be entered into a research data pool. When large data sets are available, specific statistical analysis can be performed to determine injury risk in finer detail. For example, the question of the negative effects of throwing a curveball can be better analyzed with large data sets. Other aspects of injury risk can be further quantified, such as early throwing velocity, the volume of throwing, and how it relates to injury. In addition, the features of the surgery itself, such as the type of graft used, and other variables of the surgery, can be analyzed for outcome. And, lastly, the postoperative course, the types of physical therapy performed, as well as the progression of throwing, can be fine-tuned for safest return following surgery.

EDUCATION IS OUR MOST VALUABLE WEAPON TO PREVENT INJURY

As described in Chapter 2, there are numerous myths and misperceptions of the factors that lead to injury, or the success of surgery. Education is the best method to correct these misperceptions. MLB created Pitch Smart to research and educate communities on the real risk factors. Several prominent surgeons and researchers serve on this committee, including myself. The STOP Sports Injuries program and the Baseball Health Network (baseballhealthnetwork.com) are other campaigns designed for educational opportunities to reduce injury.

SPECIFIC GUIDELINES FOR PITCH COUNTS

Understand that quality is better than quantity. Throwing fewer pitches with greater concentration and body awareness does more for developing performance and talent than huge volumes of throwing. It's much better to learn how to throw strikes by developing movement on the ball than attempting to manage velocity and the amount of break on breaking pitches.

Warm-up and Mechanics

Often, young athletes do not warm up properly. Proper warm-up before throwing in baseball playing is essential to avoid injury. It is often said you need to warm up to play catch, not play catch to warm up. Pitching should always begin with easy throws, building gradually to full effort throwing. It is common for me to hear stories about young athletes without proper throwing progression who simply go into a game to test out their arm. This occurs even after a period of rest from treatment for a specific injury. Communication must occur among parents, coaches, and players that they should not throw with pain or fatigue. This requires the athlete to take personal responsibility and feel comfortable speaking up when symptoms develop. Young pitchers should work on proper throwing mechanics even when playing simple catch.

Throwing Volume

Awareness of injury risk is essential to any parent, coach, physical therapist, or anyone involved with baseball players. The following are areas for appropriate awareness:
- Adhere to recommended pitching rules and regulations.
- Sleep and hydration are important.
- Children should be encouraged to play different sports that use different muscle groups; however, they should avoid playing multiple sports simultaneously. Pitchers should avoid swimming, tennis, and quarterbacking in football.
- Basketball in the winter is common for baseball players and is acceptable.

- A pitcher should not play catcher during the same season.
- Rest—children should rest from playing baseball for three months each year.

SIGNS AND SYMPTOMS

Never ignore symptoms of pain in a young athlete. While many coaches and parents may find regulations inhibiting to the competition and fun of baseball, it is also important to re-create a growth mind-set that injuries can be prevented, and that the fun of baseball can still be achieved and is always more fun when our kids are healthy. Encourage players to respond to signs of fatigue. If a player complains of fatigue, rest that player.

RADAR GUNS AND PERFORMANCE

Radar guns should never be used as a performance metric during adolescence. Showcases and other extended games or tournaments should be factored into the overall pitch counts of year-round and seasonal throwing and should not be excessive. Realize that premature velocity may be the biggest risk factor for injury.

GLOSSARY

Abduction: The movement of a limb away from the midline of the body.

Adduction: The movement of a limb towards the midline of the body.

Ambulation: Walking under one's own power without assistance.

Antalgic: An antalgic gait is a gait that develops as a way to avoid pain while walking (antalgic= anti- + alge, "against pain"). It is a form of gait abnormality where the stance phase of gait is abnormally shortened relative to the swing phase. It can be a good indication of pain while weight-bearing.

Atrophy: A muscular effect whereby mass is lost due to inactivity, commonly seen in the post-injury athlete.

Avulsion: A fracture that occurs, often from a strong ligamentous pull, that rather than damaging the ligament, actually pulls the ligament away from its bony insertion, with the bone fragment still intact.

Bilateral: A directional term indicating both the right and left sides of the body.

Bursa: Fluid-filled sacs that act as lubricants in joint motion between tendon and bone.

Bursitis: An inflammatory response of the bursa sac, caused by either friction or direct impact.

Closed Kinetic Chain Exercise: A form of exercise in which a limb is in contact with either the ground or other stable surface, such as a wall or table. The kinetic chain is activated with the foot or hand in contact with a surface and alters the effect of muscular action mostly by way of co-contraction.

Co-Contraction: The action of opposing muscles against one another that helps to stabilize a joint throughout its range of motion.

Commotio Codis: A sudden cardiac arrest caused by a direct blow to the chest.

Contralateral: A directional term denoting the side of the body opposite the side on which a particular injury or condition occurs; if talking about the right arm, the contralateral side is the left side.

Dermatome: An area of skin innervated by sensory fibers from a single spinal nerve.

Dislocation: Displacement of one or more bones from the supporting joint.

Distal: A directional term indicating the farthest point away from the center of the body, or away from a point of attachment.

Dorsiflexion: Ankle motion in which the foot is flexed upward toward the shin. Ex: toes to nose.

Edema: Swelling of tissue due to the body's inflammatory process.

Errythema: Redness of the skin caused by injury or infection.

Eversion: Ankle motion emanating from the subtalar joint, where the foot is extended away from the midline of the body in an outward direction.

Extensibility: A muscle or tendon's ability to be stretched.

Frontal Plane: A vertical plane that divides the body into front and back sections. Also known as the coronal plane.

Functional Exercise: An exercise that incorporates the entire body in preparation for the activities of daily life, such as squatting down and lifting an object.

Hypertrophy: An increase in muscle mass or girth through exercise.

Hypertrophic Cardiomyopathy: A sometimes fatal condition in which thickening of the heart muscle creates inefficiency pumping blood in the body.

Inferior: A directional term indicating below or underneath, or referring to the lower part of a structure or the lower of two similar structures.

Inflammatory Response: The body's natural response to injury or infection, in which blood flow is stimulated to an area to 'clean out' damaged tissue and replace with new tissue.

Inversion: Ankle motion emanating from the subtalar joint, in which the foot is extended inward toward the midline of the body.

Ipsilateral: A directional term indicating the same side of the body; if talking about the right arm, the ipsilateral side is the right side.

Jone's Fracture: A fracture at the base of the fifth metatarsal bone in the foot.

Labrum: A ring of cartilage surrounding the socket portion of both the hip and shoulder joints that acts as a smooth point of contact for motion and helps maintain the stability of the joint.

Lateral: A directional term indicating an area away from the mid-line of the body; to the side.

Ligament: A tough band of fibrous connective tissue that connects bone to bone.

Lisfranc Injury: A fracture to the bones or injury to the ligaments of the Lisfranc joint, which consists of the five bones that make up the arch in the mid-foot.

Medial: A directional term indicating an area toward the mid-line of the body.

MOI (Mechanism of Injury): The manner in which various body tissues absorb stress and are subsequently damaged. MOI is a strong indicator of what structures are likely damaged and is an important piece of information for accurate evaluation of an injury.

Mortise: The joint space at the ankle, made up of the talus, distal tibia and fibula bones.

MTBI (Mild Traumatic Brain Injury): A loss or alteration of consciousness caused by either a single impact or multiple sub-concussive impacts over time to the head.

Muscle Guarding: An immediate muscular response to an injury in which an involuntary muscular contraction acts to protect the injured limb.

Muscle Inhibition: The inability of a muscle to contract in the days following injury, caused by a loss of neuromuscular control.

Muscle Setting Exercise: A therapeutic exercise used to restore neuromuscular control to an injured limb, such as quad sets.

Open Kinetic Chain Exercise: A form of exercise in which no limbs are in contact with a stable surface, such as the ground or a wall or table. The kinetic chain is activated in an open-ended manner and alters the effect of muscular action on a joint by decreasing joint compressive forces and eliminating co-contraction.

Periodization: Systematic planning of athletic or physical training. The goal is to reach optimal performance at some critical time, e.g., playoffs, tryouts. It requires progressive cycling in a training program.

Pes Cavus: A foot shape with a pronounced arch and increased supination; a high in-step.

Pes Planus: A foot shape with essentially no arch, with the medial foot in contact with the ground; flat-footed.

Plantarflexion: Ankle motion in which the toes are pointed downward toward the ground.

Platelet-Rich Plasma (PRP) Injection: A method of therapy in which an individual's own blood is spun in a centrifuge to remove the dense plasma, which is then injected directly into the site of musculoskeletal injury to promote healing.

PRE (Progressive Resistive Exercises): An exercise plan in which a foundation is formed prior to increasing weights or resistance.

Prone: A body position in which an individual lies face down on the floor or table.

Proprioception: The body's awareness of a joint or limb's relative position in time and space.

Proximal: A directional term indicating the closest point toward the center of the body, or closer to a point of attachment.

Range of Motion: The distance a joint can move between the flexed position and the extended position.

Retinaculum: Thin, fibrous bands of connective tissue that encapsulate groups of tendons around the joints and hold them in place.

Sagittal Plane: The vertical plane that passes from front to back, dividing the body into right and left halves.

Sport-Specific Exercise: Any exercise designed to mimic the demands of a particular sport or position.

Sprain: A ligamentous injury, often resulting from overstretching the tissue, ranging in severity from Grades 1 to 3.

Strain: A musculotendinous injury, often resulting from overstretching the tissue, ranging in severity from Grades 1 to 3.

Subluxation: An incomplete or partial dislocation.

Superior: A directional term indicating above, on top of, or towards the head.

Supine: A body position in which an individual is lying flat on the floor or a table with the face up.

Syndesmosis: An articulation, allowing for a minimal range of motion, in which two bones are connected.

Tendon: A tough band of fibrous connective tissue that connects muscle to bone.

Tendinitis: An inflammatory response within a tendon or tendon sheath which results in pain and loss of function.

Transverse Plane: A horizontal plane that divides the body in half from top to bottom, perpendicular to the sagittal and frontal planes.

Valgus Stress: Stress applied to any joint that is directed in a lateral to medial manner and stretches tissue on the medial (inside) aspect of the joint.

Varus Stress: Stress applied to any joint directed in a medial to lateral manner that stretches tissue on the lateral (outside) aspect of the joint.

ABOUT THE AUTHORS

Christopher S. Ahmad, MD, specializes in ACL knee injuries, meniscus and cartilage injuries, instability and labral tears of the shoulder, rotator cuff pathology, Tommy John surgery, and advanced arthroscopic surgical techniques for sports-related injuries of the knee, shoulder, and elbow. Dr. Ahmad is the Head Team Physician for the New York Yankees, the Rockland Boulders, the New York City Football Club of Major League Soccer, and several high schools throughout Manhattan and New Jersey. Additionally, he is a member of the Major League Baseball Team Physicians Association, serves as a consultant for local metropolitan gymnastics and swim teams, and is the official medical provider to the FC Westchester Soccer Academy.

The recipient of several awards for outstanding research in the field of Sports Medicine, Dr. Ahmad conducts ongoing research in the areas of ACL injury prevention and screening, biometrics of the elbow, and surgical techniques for rotator cuff shoulder instability repair. He has authored more than 200 articles and 50 book chapters related to shoulder, elbow and sports medicine and has presented over 250 lectures nationally, and internationally. Dr. Ahmad edited two influential textbooks: *Minimally Invasive Shoulder and Elbow Surgery* and *Pediatric and Adolescent Sports Injuries.*

He earned his undergraduate degree in engineering while playing four years of Division 1 varsity soccer at nationally ranked Columbia University. I Ie lives in Manhattan with his wife and three children.

John Gallucci, Jr., MS, ATC, PT, DPT, the dynamic President and CEO of JAG Physical Therapy, is in demand for his expertise in injury prevention, rehabilitation, sports medicine, and athletic conditioning. He has appeared often on radio and television, including ESPN's award-winning *Outside the Lines*, MSG Varsity, NJ News 12, and WFAN. Gallucci is a popular public speaker.

Gallucci has made a major impact in his fields throughout the New York/New Jersey area, and holds a national presence in the sports medicine community. JAG Physical Therapy now offers comprehensive orthopedic outpatient centers in West Orange, Warren, Cedar Knolls, Union, Hackensack, Woodbridge, Fairfield, Old Bridge, Holmdel, Chatham, Brick, Wayne, and Princeton, New Jersey, as well as Sleepy Hollow, Yonkers, Hawthorne, and New York, NY.

Currently, John is the Medical Coordinator for Major League Soccer (MLS), coordinating the medical care of more than 500 professional soccer players. Gallucci is the former Head Athletic Trainer of the New York Red Bulls MLS team and is a Sports Medicine consultant for professional athletes in the NHL, NFL, NBA, MLB, and USA Wrestling. John has also worked in the Athletic Departments of Columbia University, New York University, and Long Island University, as well as being a Clinical Instructor at Columbia University, Seton Hall University, Rutgers University, and Dominican College. John is the former Program Director of Barnabas Health's Sport Medicine Institute and also serves as the Chair of the New Jersey Council on Physical Fitness and Sports.

In June 2017, John was named an Ernst & Young Entrepreneur of the Year Regional Award Winner, known as the world's most prestigious business awards program for entrepreneurs. In addition, John has been recognized as a two-time Smart CEO Future 50 Award Winner, 2016 NJ Biz Healthcare Heroes Education Hero Award Winner, and was featured by *201 Magazine* as one of "20 People to Watch in Health" in 2016. In addition, JAG Physical Therapy is honored to be the most awarded physical therapy company in the Tri-State Area, including being recognized as the Physical Therapy Company of the Year by *NJBIZ*.